Cats are mysterious and unpredictable—
but if you learn to understand your
cat's instincts, you can also understand
his behavior. Animal expert Mordecai
Siegal explains the causes of common
cat misbehaviors—and offers simple
solutions for . . .

- AGGRESSIVENESS
- TIMIDITY
- DESTRUCTIVE BEHAVIOR
- CONFLICTS WITH OTHER PETS

- AND MORE

UNDERSTANDING THE CAT YOU LOVE

Berkley Books by Mordecai Siegal

HAPPY KITTENS, HAPPY CATS
YOUR NEW BEST FRIEND
UNDERSTANDING THE DOG YOU LOVE
UNDERSTANDING THE CAT YOU LOVE

UNDERSTANDING THE CAT YOU LOVE

MORDECAI SIEGAL

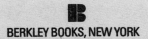

BERKLEY BOOKS, NEW YORK

UNDERSTANDING THE CAT YOU LOVE

A Berkley Book / published by arrangement with the author

PRINTING HISTORY
Berkley edition / December 1994

ISBN: 0-425-14498-4

BERKLEY®
Berkley Books are published by
The Berkley Publishing Group, 200 Madison Avenue,
New York, New York 10016.
BERKLEY and the "B" design are trademarks of
Berkley Publishing Corporation.

PRINTED IN THE UNITED STATES OF AMERICA

10 9 8 7 6 5 4 3 2 1

To my dear friend Harry Paine,
who has always had a tender place
in his heart for cats

CONTENTS

INTRODUCTION

"A cat times nine" is simply one of many myths. Our feline friends are not now, nor have they ever been, furry gods or magical beings with supernatural powers. They are not all-knowing, all-seeing and all-powerful. Rather, cats are living, breathing creatures like us and as such are subject to the many spins of life's wheel of fortune. In between mewing and meowing and warming our hearts by leaping into our laps, they also get sick, become upset, caterwaul, shred our furniture with their claws, run around till all hours of the night, and totally dominate our lives. It is definitely *not* a good idea to imagine the cat of your dreams to be a white puff of fur with a large, red satin bow tied around its neck as it merrily jumps out of a half-empty chocolate box. That image will evaporate instantly for the new cat owner immediately after cleaning a used litter pan or experiencing a male cat spraying sexually scented urine on a wall to proclaim his territory.

There is more to cats than the romantic images found on old birthday cards and bookmarkers. Nowadays everyone understands that cats, like dogs, are companion animals that do their job with consummate skill. They represent one of the few fragments of nature left to us in our society of cement and aluminum city parks and planned parking suburbs. Cats, no matter how confined within the four walls of our homes, are carpet-bound microcosms of nature in the wild, as they display their primitive behavior at catnip mice and rolling Ping-Pong balls.

This book is about learning to live with the best behaved cat possible. But what does that mean? Is the best behaved cat the one that obeys you the instant you give it a command? Not really. That is an impractical desire because cats do not respond to human demands the way dogs do. The best cats are the ones who please you the most, and that has a lot to do with behavior and misbehavior.

Your cat's behavior is the most important aspect of a successful human-pet relationship. The natural behavior of cats is compatible, for the most part, with the way humans live, if it is understood and dealt with properly. Although cats are solitary creatures in their wild or natural state, they do develop deep and lasting relationships with humans if given the chance. This is part of what makes them so endearing. Understanding natural cat behavior helps pet owners cope with feline housebreaking problems, destructive behavior, noisy meowing through the night, and the other upsetting things that cats like to do. Learning what goes on inside your cat's mind will help to create the bond that is so desirable between humans and their pets. Once the bond is established, new cats become members of the family and bring out loving instincts that make most new cat owners parents, pals, or partners.

Because we feel so deeply about our cats, we tend to think of them as humans. We interpret their every move as human behavior rather than cat behavior, from looking us directly in the eyes to patting us on the arm with their paws when they want to be fed. All pet owners are like this, from presidents to movie stars to everyone who ever showed off photos of the family pet. The fact is, however, there is such a thing as *natural* cat behavior, and it is quite different from *human* behavior. If you understand the difference, you can prevent many behavior problems from developing and manage most of those that are already present. All cats, no matter how they live with humans, are born with a set of natural behavior patterns that are exclusively feline. Some of them blend in perfectly with ours and some do not. This is true of house pets, show cats, and every feline that ever crept into our hearts.

When considering the quality of cats, one cannot ignore the distinctions between *pet owners* and *cat fanciers*. Although they often cross lines, these two groups are involved in different ways. The differences are important.

Pet owners think of their cats as members of the family. How they treat their cats depends on how they treat their families. Pet cats are expected to give and receive love and companionship in exchange for kind treatment, a full belly, and a warm place to sleep. Some pets are four-legged love objects and are smothered with affection, food, and constant attention. Some pets are treated like rich relatives. Their misbehavior is either ignored or regarded as endearing and simply tolerated no matter what. However, the typical family cat risks losing the love of his family when his behavior becomes unacceptable or unbearable. Most pet cats cannot escape the consequences of their own unacceptable behavior unless their human benefactors learn how to change it or cope with it.

Cat fanciers, on the other hand, have a professional interest and expect more than companionship and member-of-the-family status. They are the breeders, exhibitors, show judges, veterinarians, professional groomers, writers, and connoisseurs of the feline arts, sciences, and sports. Although many fanciers relate to their cats as pets, they are also concerned with every aspect of the cat world, including professional health care, competition in cat shows, and attempting to achieve breed perfection according to standards set forth by various cat clubs and associations.

Serious cat fanciers, especially breeders, judges, and exhibitors are, in a practical sense, historians and stewards of the many cat breeds that exist today. They are part of an effort to preserve (and possibly improve) the best physical and mental qualities of the various cat breeds. They help to create and preserve breed standards by which individual cats are measured for their look, temperament, and function. The principles of genetics, animal husbandry, and good cat handling are necessary to achieve their goals.

Purebred cats must be carefully selected for their best characteristics before they are allowed to mate. They must measure up to the standard created for each of their respective breeds. Temperamentally unstable, physically impaired, or seriously flawed examples of a breed are usually rejected for breeding by conscientious cat fanciers. The goal of very serious breeders is to produce healthy kittens that grow into beautiful cats. Their cats must represent the standard of their breed as set forth by a national breed club and adopted by such organizations as the Cat Fanciers' Association, the American Cat Association, or one of the other national cat organizations that register purebred cats in the United States and Canada. As you can see, the differences between cat fanciers and pet owners are great.

Unless you want to compete at cat shows or begin a serious breeding program, your cat's "papers," CFA or otherwise, have no value except to keep the floor clean. It is not important if your cat is a pure breed or a mixed breed, a movie star or a house cat. The most important consideration is that your cat is compatible with you, enjoyable, and under control. For pet owners the best cats are not necessarily Grand Champions or blue ribbon winners.

The best cats are the ones that are healthy, happy, easy to love, who have entered your lives and altered your capacity for change while teaching you something about your feelings.

This book is about understanding cats and how to make life better for them and the people who love them. It deals with what is acceptable and unacceptable cat behavior and realistic and unrealistic human expectations. It is a practical book that offers solutions to some problems through an informal understanding of why cats are the way they are.

UNDERSTANDING THE CAT YOU LOVE

KITTEN DAZE

It may come as a surprise, but your sweet adorable kitten is more like his wild cousins in the jungles, mountains, and deserts than the dog is like its cousin, the wolf. That is why it is important to understand the nature of your little furry tiger and recognize what is going on when he attacks your big toe or plays havoc with whatever is lying around your house at night. The cat has never been as domesticated as the dog. Dogs instinctively live in social structures of their own (packs). Human families easily substitute for dog packs. But almost all cats live a solitary existence in the wild and therefore are not genetically programmed to live with other creatures, whether they are other cats or human substitutes. It is only after thousands of generations of domestication, adaptation, and human bribery that cats have gone against their most primitive instincts to go it alone. Most house cats live as solitary an existence as circumstances will allow.

In their natural state, cats must hunt for a living, carve out a territory, mate, and fight for all of these accomplishments when necessary. These abilities are partially inherited, partially taught by the mother cat's example and instruction, and partially learned from the behavior of litter mates. In the wild the motivation behind the cat's behavior is hunger, sex, fear, or anxiety. To this, add a highly qualified form of affection and dependency, and you have a fairly complete picture of the domestic feline temperament, from kitten to adult cat.

Kitten Development

You do not have to be a behavioral scientist to understand that if a kitten is taken from its mother and its litter mates too soon, is denied physical contact with others, is isolated, or lives in a state of fear, it will probably have severe behavioral problems throughout its life. It will either be too shy or too aggressive or too something. Behavior researchers have established this predictable pattern. Most parents have known this for generations with regard to their own children.

The ideal cat grows from a kitten that is adaptive, social, curious, playful, and unafraid of new experiences and people (within limits). As with most mammals, especially domestic animals and humans, early experiences in infancy and childhood have a profound influence on the individual cat's temperament and behavior.

The first week of life. All kittens are born without teeth. Their eyes are sealed shut and their ears are folded down. They cannot see, hear, or eat solid food. They can barely move. Body weight is between three and five ounces.

For the first few days the kittens are unable to move away from their mother and consequently lie close to her for warmth and food. Becoming chilled is the greatest threat to their lives. The first week of their lives involves staying warm, nursing, and sleeping. They can do little more than sense their mother's warm body by touch and smell.

Taking breast milk usually begins by the first or second hour of life and is started with the mother's urging. During the initial period of rapid growth healthy kittens will gain weight at the rate of approximately a half an ounce a day. Kittens double their birth weight by seven days and triple it by twenty-one days, with males gaining a little more. Rapid growth continues for approximately six to twelve months, adding close to one pound every four weeks.

By the second day each kitten claims one of Mother's nipples and a kind of ownership develops. For every feeding, the kitten returns to the claimed nipple, which is found by the establishment of a scent around it. This is the beginning of behavior based on territorial claims and boundaries and facilitated by the use of personal odors, which has a profound influence on the cat's behavior throughout his life.

For almost the entire first three weeks of life the newborns are unable to eliminate urine and feces on their own. They must rely on their mother for stimulation of the digestive system. She must frequently lick the genital areas of each kitten in order to promote elimination. In the process she keeps the nest clean by ingesting their body waste. Her primary responsibilities are to keep the kittens warm, fed, and in one place despite the fact that they tend to "waddle" away from her with their forepaws. The mother retrieves missing kittens by the sound of their high-pitched mewing, which they are capable of emitting almost from birth.

The second week. At this stage life continues in a shadowy world of muted sounds. Only the sense of warmth, cold, hunger, and bodily contact with the mother and litter mates lets the kittens know that they are alive. Their eyes and ears begin the process of developing, but just barely. The process takes approximately three days. Movement within the nest is a bit more active. Their voices are louder and stronger. Nursing behavior during this period continues to be initiated by the mother.

The third week. Up until this time the mother had to encourage the kittens to nurse. By approximately the twentieth day the kittens themselves initiate nursing by following the mother around and meowing insistently to be fed.

At this time the kittens crawl around swiftly and are beginning to stand, although they are wobbly. Their eyes have opened fully and their ears are straightening. The kittens can now see, hear, and walk. Tiny teeth emerge in preparation for eating solid food. Individual personalities begin to develop, and the kittens take on a more catlike appearance rather than the formless shapes they were. It is now possible to determine male from female by observing the genitalia. Although there are no signs of learning, they respond to their mother's movements and seem to be experiencing sensory, motor, and psychological changes. They become very active and climb out of the nest to explore, much to the mother's disapproval. Play behavior between litter mates and some tolerant mothers begins during this period. It takes the form of pretended aggressiveness, wrestling, pouncing, and swatting with the paws.

Four to eight weeks. Weaning from Mother's milk to solid food begins or has already begun at this time. The complete transition to solid food is usually accomplished by six to eight weeks of age with the mother cat resisting or refusing to nurse the kittens. The kittens can now stand and feed from a bowl.

Play is now seen in full swing, and self-grooming has become a permanent set of behaviors. Kittens at this age usually weigh more than two pounds, are quite robust, and possess a full set of sharp teeth. They are well on the road to full growth and maturity.

Social Development

Although the rigors of scientific research have been applied to the behavior and critical stages of social development for puppies and dogs, little has been done in this area with cats. What *is* known has come from the practical experience of conscientious breeders who were influenced by the conclusions drawn about kitten development based on puppy development.

With puppies the critical stage for social development is between the third and twelfth week of life. What happens during this period sets a pattern for all future behavior. It is this stage when socialization begins and the puppies form relationships with human beings and other animals. Researchers have suggested that each puppy at this time be removed daily from the litter for a short time and brought into contact with human beings. The puppies should be handled and cuddled lovingly several times a day. This process of socialization, enables a dog to realize his maximum potential as a domestic house pet and companion as well as the ability to adjust happily to other animals.

Many cat experts have recommended that similar attention be paid to kittens. Some have even suggested that handling begin as soon as possible during the first thirty days of life, to produce a more adaptive, more social, and less fearful cat.

Young kittens should be given toys and various household objects to play with such as sewing spools, paper bags, cardboard boxes, etc. in order to stimulate early learning and physical development. Young kittens should be exposed to a variety of people, places and things to avoid timid, fearful cats who shun most humans and new experiences. In this way, it is possible to shape your kitten's personality.

The Playful Kitten

Cats have a bad press when it comes to love, dependency, and expressions of affection. Don't you believe it, especially when it comes to kittens. Despite his devilishly impish behavior there is nothing more affectionate (and playful) than a kitten that has made his adjustment to your home. Although baby cats are capable of amusing themselves for hours on end, they would almost all rather engage you, the pet owner, in their frisky romps around the house. As a play/learning experience, they will attack your shoelaces with great energy. They will jump in your lap like a mountain lion springing from the limb of a tree to catch a four-legged meal. A learning kitten is usually fearless. That is what makes it so amusing (and so accident prone).

Actually, there is nothing more demanding than a kitten looking up at its human family, wanting to be held and petted. Yes, kittens and many adult cats crave loving affection just like other pets. Kittens, however, are the needle-toothed jumping jacks of the order *Carnivora*. They cannot sit still for more than a few seconds and are constantly clawing your thighs or your arms for traction to launch themselves to the next object of play.

The primary activity of kittenhood is learning to survive in a wild state. (Nature never took into account the doting cat owner or compensated for the efficient pet food industry.) Kittens learn to survive through the activity of play. Although it is comical and heartwarming to watch a litter of kittens hard at play, what you are witnessing is a lesson in fighting, hunting, and escape maneuvers.

Assuming that most play behavior in cats is a form of learning relevant to catching a meal (for the sake of survival), then we can only imagine that different techniques in play are meant to teach how to capture different kinds of prey. Catching a bird, for example, is far more difficult than catching a mouse, and requires learning different techniques. If a kitten hears something that sounds like a chirp from above, it instinctively looks up and tries to develop a jumping technique for capturing the aerial source of provocative noise. Hence, a lamp may fall because it was in the path of some higher source of sound.

Nothing is more fascinating than watching a grown cat after a moth or a fly. It simply follows the flying object around for a long time before it makes any aggressive move. The cat is studying the pattern of takeoff, flight, and landing so that it can predict where the fly will go next. This is the same principle used in catching mice. Mousing is somewhat easier for a cat because the rodent usually moves along prescribed paths and routes and does not have enough time to adapt its plan to take into consideration the feline predator waiting at the point of entry or exit. Some cats simply wait at the mouse hole, sometimes for hours, knowing full well that the tiny creature will appear and be taken. But all this is hard-earned information learned primarily through play behavior as a kitten.

Kittens that are held by humans and are given toys at an early age to awaken their sense of play usually grow into happy, intelligent creatures. Whatever the potential of the cat, it can be best achieved through early affection and stimulation. Toys are very important because they stimulate and provoke play. Kitten play in the early life of a cat is the equivalent of grade school for a child.

Although play is an important means of exercise for

domestic cats, it is primarily a learning and practicing process for activities connected with survival. Obviously the need for survival techniques no longer exists for pampered house cats, but genetic programming has not caught up with the realities of pet life. The tendency to learn the techniques of survival is strong and to some extent genetically organized. Whether the cat ever really learns the specifics is quite another matter. Some cats chase mice and others do not. Some will fight while others acquiesce. These specific behaviors are determined by early education from the mother and litter mates, as are other behaviors pertaining to dominance and subordination, mating, gender, and territory.

What a kitten is rehearsing during play is a drama of survival fighting, sexual behavior, territorial defense, and all those activities connected with hunting, which include tracking, trailing, stalking, capturing prey, and the killing and eating of prey animals. In kittens, however, what begins as a serious drama always turns into a howling good comedy.

Kitten Toys

When selecting toys for kittens and grown cats, try to get something that will provoke the various activities described above. For example, the single most attractive toy for a cat is a Ping-Pong ball. It is small like a mouse, it moves in quick, unpredictable motions, and it has a spectacular sound when bounced. In other words, many senses and instinctive responses are called into play. Try dropping a walnut or small rubber ball into an empty tissue box and giving it to your cat as a toy. The cat will regard the object as a mouse and manipulate it with both paws.

The toys most frequently purchased for cats in stores

are little felt mice, generally advertised as catnip mice. The truth of the matter is that many of these items do not contain catnip at all. They are sprayed with some substance of fleeting interest to the cat, and filled with some chopped plant or tree bark that resembles catnip. Without true catnip the toy is merely an expensive colored piece of felt that will probably just lie there while your cat pursues a plain piece of paper or a brown paper bag with much more relish. Cats do enjoy felt mice that contain real catnip.

A string or a rope is a good toy as long as you hold one end and work it like a snake. Put it safely away when you're not around to prevent your pet from swallowing it. Be careful of toys with metal whistles or bells, sharp objects, or small buttons. A cat toy should be safe and not have on it anything that can be swallowed.

Peacock feathers are wonderful; they offer movement, shape, and texture. Waving the feather before the kitten's eyes in a bouncing motion, tickling the nose and feet— all such activities stimulate the hunter in your cat and will divert the animal for quite a while. Hard rubber balls, large sewing spools, or almost anything that rolls make excellent toys. Containers such as cardboard boxes, large pots, paper bags, straw hats, or even wastebaskets appeal to a cat's inherent need to practice hiding and escaping.

Some scratch posts come equipped with a rubber ball attached to the top by an elastic string. These can be great fun and often keep the cat's interest focused on the scratch post instead of your furniture, and isn't that a good thing. The finest cat toy available, the one that offers the most play (if you will play too), is a crumpled sheet of paper.

Cats are nocturnal creatures who hunt, mate, and work out territory in the dark. Kittens play at these activities through the night hours and cannot help themselves.

The Needful Kitten

Because of the thousands of years of domestication, there are some major differences between house cats and those living in the wild. A cat living by itself in the wild is somewhat paranoid in its behavior and would fear every move made by any strange creature, including human beings. Even though domestic cats have the capacity to revert instantly to wild behavior when they have to, and always live within a shadow of their own wild behavior, there are still dependencies that have developed. Kittens adjust or socialize to human handling and kindness and shift their dependency easily from a mother cat to a human benefactor. For these reasons, kittens may feel reassured in the dark by the sounds of their human family tossing and turning in their beds, even from the sounds of snoring.

Once patterns are established early in a cat's life, it is almost impossible to break them. Somebody opens a can of cat food. Somebody changes the litter pan. The cat becomes accustomed to these services very quickly in the game. In one day a kitten may attach itself to its owner, whose need of the cat may become as great as the kitten's need of him or her. It is a bonding process that works both ways. Once a person kisses a kitten, cuddles it, hugs it, feeds it, contact has been made between two beings and attachments develop. Kittens are too young and too small and too dependent to be on their own in the wild or to reject the protection of the human situation.

If a cat coming into a new home has been on its own for a long period of time, it becomes very difficult to achieve an adjustment to the traditional pet life style. Such a cat or kitten might concentrate all its efforts on escaping back into the wild. But a normal kitten wants to be taken care of and to be made secure. Domesticity in pets is probably based on humans' constant appeal to the infant and adolescent aspect of the animal's nature. And so, to hear the family sleeping upstairs is to know that the family is there and that everything is safe despite the newness of the situation.

Play is a serious business for a kitten, or even some adult cats, but that is something the human family must learn. A few hours of lost sleep in the beginning of a kitten-human relationship is to be expected and well worth the trouble.

Kitten Proofing Your Home

• It is imperative that your new kitten not be allowed to get out of the house. There is nothing more curious than a kitten in a new home. Curiosity *can* kill a cat. Check your living space for avenues of escape such as holes, broken doors, faulty screens, or open windows. This is especially important for apartment dwellers living in tall buildings. A two- to three-inch opening is all that's necessary for a kitten (or a grown cat) to squeeze through. The great outdoors is no place for a grown cat, much less a defenseless kitten.

• Allow no opportunity for the kitten to fall into water. If you own a swimming pool, do not let the little cat out of the house for a minute.

• Keep the lid of the toilet down. Never leave a kitten near a tub unless the stopper is out and the water is drained. The same applies for washing machines, sinks, and pails. Speaking of washing machines, always close the door to the electric clothes dryer. A tumble-dried kitten is neither fluffy nor amusing. It is a common accident that results in death.

• Take a walk around your premises and look for dangling cords, wires, ropes, shade pulls, venetian blind strings, fishing tackle, vacuum cleaner tubes, TV antenna cable, and even leather thongs on pot handles. They all appeal to a young cat as devices for exercise and play. But they all represent hidden death traps for a frisky mischief maker.

• Put dangerous objects away. Fold up excess cords and tape them to a wall or under a table. Bits of yarn, string, and ribbon are easily swallowed and can cause intestinal blockages, constipation, and various stomach ailments. Keep this material off the floor and tables.

• Electrical cords are a double dose of trouble. A kitten is likely to attack a dangling wire and pull down the appliance on top of himself. This can happen with toasters, blenders, electric frying pans (while in use), coffeepots, and juicers. If the youngster is not scalded or brained, he could be electrocuted by plunging his tiny razorlike teeth into the wire. This is true of any electric device with a wire plugged into a wall receptacle.

• Often without knowing it, owners of every household maintain a well-stocked supply of poisons. Many household cleaners are poisonous to humans as well as to animals. Small animals and children are especially vulnerable to common poisons because small doses can make them seriously ill. Poisons kittens most commonly get into include lead (as in paints, ceramics, paperweights), petroleum distillates (such as kerosene), detergents, lye, cleansers, mothballs, insecticides, and all medications, including aspirin, sleeping pills, tranquilizers, and various cold remedies.

• It goes without saying that controlled substances such as drugs used by humans are lethal in most cases for small animals (and children). Methadone, LSD, marijuana, heroin, amphetamines, and all the various things that are sniffed, from cocaine to glue, can kill a kitten or grown cat. It is bad enough to have an animal get at them through carelessness, but it is a cruel and an inhumane crime to feed drugs purposely to an animal.

• Keep your kitten out of your garage or basement, where it might get into antifreeze and all the other poisonous fluids used for your automobile. Antifreeze has an attractive color and sweet taste. Cats, dogs, and even small children are attracted to it. They will lick it off the floor if given the opportunity. Antifreeze will cause death.

• Some plants are poisonous, and this should be looked into when bringing a kitten into your house.

• If there are children in the house, they must be made aware of the dangers caused by some of their toys. Bicycles, tricycles, skateboards, roller blades, and all other toys with wheels represent a potential hazard.

• Do not leave any plastic bags lying around for the kitten to get into. All plastic bags can cause immediate suffocation.

• Before you close your refrigerator door, make sure the kitten hasn't jumped in.

• Never allow the kitten to be around during the operation of any machinery, from the vacuum cleaner to the lawn mower to the radio-operated garage door.

• Screen off your fireplace lest your roaming cat attempt to climb up the chimney.

• Remove your breakables from table surfaces and countertops.

• Cover the top of your aquarium.

• Elevate the height of your bird cage.

• Keep the hamsters and gerbils in secure cages and place them in a room the kitten cannot enter.

• Cover all trash cans.

• Close all drawers, cupboards, closets, appliances, and medicine cabinets.

Sooner or later every cat gets into trouble. Watch your kitten until he settles down in his new home, and even then, be vigilant.

First Impressions

When a young kitten comes to live with you for the first time, it is an exciting, delightful experience . . . for a while. But the realities of this living, breathing life form confront the novice cat owner with the challenge of coping with strange, new behaviors that are far different from human actions and responses. The seemingly shy reticence displayed by a new kitten is in sharp contrast to its sudden darts of energy as it leaps from your lap to your shoulder to the top of your furniture. Kittens run, hide, jump, pounce, nip, claw, chase, and then act timid, tired, or tyranical. They are unpredictable, and also impressionable. The early hours, days, and weeks with a new kitten help determine the nature of your relationship and how the kitten will behave in your home.

It is easy for new cat owners to fail in their relationships with the new family pet because of what happens at this very important time. The kitten is led into the house like a prize lion entering the Colosseum to the cheers of a thrill-seeking mob falling all over itself in a deluge of mass hysteria. It is a great mistake to introduce a kitten into its new home in this fashion. A kitten's earliest experiences have a lasting effect on its behavior and mental hygiene.

A kitten is essentially an infant or very young animal of about seven to twelve weeks of age, perhaps leaving its mother and litter mates for the first time to enter the society of humans. All that was warm, secure, and known is gone, evaporated with the closing of the flaps of a cardboard carton. The kitten's world has suddenly and without warning expanded to unmanageable proportions inhabited by large, vertical creatures stripping it of all choice and freedom. These mammoth two-legged monsters reach down from the heights and grab and clutch and squeeze while uttering the most terrifying, unbeautiful sounds. We are then left with a fear-ridden, overexcited victim with no means of escape or ability to adapt. The result may be the start of abnormal behavior which, in human terms, is called neurosis. The early experiences of kittens could create shyness, aggressiveness, or combinations of both. This is not fair. It is not necessary.

Making an Entrance

When you first enter your home with a new kitten, your objective is to complete the disturbing transition for the little cat with as little trauma and overstimulation as possible. It is certainly impossible to bring a kitten into a house where children live and deprive them of meeting the new member of the family. This applies to the adult residents as well. In order to satisfy this urgent need, you may offer a quick but gratifying peek. Devote five minutes for quick introductions and one or two *calm* strokes on the cat's body. Make it clear that the family—especially the children—are not to stimulate the kitten with loud squeals, giggles, hugs, kisses, or other physicalized or overly vocalized expressions of delight. Remember, it's the cat we are concerned with at this moment. After the brief time allotted for introductions, chase the family into another part of the house for at least an hour and perhaps the rest of the day.

Noise

Arrange with your family and visitors to keep the noise level to a bare minimum. Loud sounds interfere with the kitten's ability to accept the new environment as his own. Loud radios, televisions, phonographs, or the frantic squeals of playful children will scare a new kitten. They will make it more difficult for the kitten to adjust to your home and to his new family. A subdued environment, peace and quiet, and low-key lighting help toward that end and are suggested for the first hour or two with your new kitten.

A Friendly Voice

It is impossible to predict how the new kitten will feel at this point in his journey. It depends on the kitten's personality, his breed characteristics, the way he's been handled in the first weeks of his life, and many other variables. The kitten may have been quite frisky when you got him but is now wilted or dejected from the great change. The most sensible goal for the new owner is to gain the cat's confidence. You have already begun by keeping the introductions short, lowering the noise level, subduing the lighting, and not forcing the kitten to relate to anyone other than yourself. And this brings us to the question of how you can relate to the cat so that he will trust you and his new surroundings.

This has to do with communication. Everything you do or say has an effect on the cat. Ideally, you want to do and say those things that communicate safety, affection, and comfort to the baby cat. This is accomplished by avoiding sudden moves around the kitten, especially those motions that are directed toward the cat. Move slowly and smoothly and do not grab or clutch. Although most cats come to understand some words, they don't at this stage of their lives. Your kitten will respond positively to a soothing, gentle tone of voice, however. Do not be inhibited about talking to your cat. You will eventually do it anyway. You may experience direct communication at this early point if you start talking in a soft, friendly manner. Once you gain your cat's confidence, you will have it all the cat's life—providing you don't abuse the cat. Having a cat's confidence means you will have little difficulty in shaping him into the kind of friend and companion you want.

How to Hold Your Cat

From a new kitten's point of view he is in danger, or at least in a state of anxiety caused by the uncertainty of his strange situation. He doesn't know where he is or who these creatures are and whether they are going to bring harm or not. It is your job to convince this animal that he is in good hands.

Avoid holding a cat in any way that scares the animal. The cat may panic and try to squirm away, and in the process you may be severely scratched or the cat may have a bad fall. This is easily avoided when you know how to pick the cat up.

Slide your hand along the belly and up to the chest; stop when your fingers are just behind the front legs. Place the cat's rear end and back legs in the open palm of your other hand. Be firm but gentle and it will be almost impossible to lose the animal.

Investigating His New Home

With no one but yourself in the immediate area, allow the cat to take a look and a sniff at the new home. Instead of giving the kitten the complete run of the house, take him into one room at a time, allowing him to see the entire territory and range. But do not let the newcomer roam too far away from you. It is especially useful to show the kitten the food bowl first. Place a small quantity of high-quality cat food in the dish or an appealing morsel such as bits of cooked liver or some commercial snack product. Have a bowl of water waiting in the place where it will always be. After this take the kitten in your arms and to the location of the litter pan and place the kitten in it. The young cat may or may not know what to do in it, but that will come later. Please refer to Chapter Six, "How To Train Your Cat." Allow the kitten to roam around at will, making sure to follow him wherever he chooses to go. Just be patient.

It is now time for the first feeding. Get out the food and place it in the bowl or dish. Do not bring the food to the cat; do it the other way around. This is the time to establish desirable habits. Show the cat where to eat and drink, where his toilet is, the scratch post, and where he is to sleep.

By the way, it is a good idea to select the cat's name right away and to begin using it immediately. Naming a cat is such a subjective matter that it hardly bears mentioning. No matter what elaborate or comical or literary name you choose, have a one-syllable call-name in addition, because that is the one you will probably use most of the time. Pets learn one-syllable names quickly and respond best to them.

The First Day

On the first day, nothing more than an introduction to the family and to those areas pertaining to the kitten should be emphasized. Feed, water, and toilet the animal. Allow the cat to explore one room at a time. Keep him away from other household pets and children (if possible), and then give him some rest. Talk to him gently and use his name as often as you can. Do not play with the cat too energetically. Do not take the animal outdoors and do not bring any friends or neighbors in to see the newcomer. A sedate, restful environment is best for the first day.

It is quite likely that your new kitten is going to go directly under a sofa and hide for a while. You will need to tolerate this; regard it as an expression of anxiety, not a personal rejection. It is natural for all cats to seek a dark, safe spot when they think they might be in danger.

Do not move the furniture or force the situation in any way. You might make some very gentle, playful sounds and gestures. Let the animal hide, if he insists, until mealtime. You might have to offer some food on your finger as an enticement to come out. If he accepts the food, get him to follow you to his feeding area (or carry him there). Be relaxed and soothing in your tone and manner. After he has eaten, take him to the litter pan, and from there to his bed for a nap. If the kitten insists on hiding under the sofa, be patient. He will venture out sooner or later.

Night Falls

Cats are nocturnal creatures who hunt, mate, and work out territorial matters in the dark. Kittens play at these activities through the night hours and cannot help themselves. The first night with a kitten can be upsetting if you are not prepared for what might happen. You may find yourself awakened by a constant, unrelenting mewing and meowing, or you may be disturbed by running back and forth, frantic scratching sounds, or even the thud of an object falling to the floor. Your trash pail may be knocked over or a lamp may be rolling on the floor, with your surprised kitten looking up at you wondering why you are upset, as he scampers into the darkness. Sometimes this continues throughout the night unless you confine the cat to one place, although that does not guarantee he will not scratch at the door continually or continue to cry out.

The first week with your new cat will probably be more

difficult at night. This is a time for adjustment to the new home coupled with activities related to the growth and development of young kittens. It is the most difficult time for the first-time cat owner. It is also a time, however, when kittens are the most charming, the most humorous, and the most endearing. All cat owners have funny stories about the first nights spent with their cats.

If you remove a kitten from his litter mates, his mother, and his familiar surroundings, he is going to be disoriented and anxious. Even a kitten from a pet shop is going to need time to make the transition from one environment to another. You must have faith in the certainty that your cat will soon adjust to his new home and allow you to get a night's sleep.

Once patterns are established early in a kitten's life, it is almost impossible to break them. A kitten is too young to be off on its own in the wild or in your house. In a very short time he will not only accept the generosity of your protection, he will demand it.

One way to cope with the nocturnal activities of a new kitten is to confine the animal to one room for the night. The best place is where the food, water, scratch post, and litter pan are located. The only problem with this is the cat's anxiety. Some kittens will adjust to being confined in one room alone for the night and some will not (for a while, anyway). You can choose to confine the kitten in your room (with the door closed) if you do not mind his sleeping with you in the bed, because that is where he will go. Take the new cat bed in with you and place it on the floor and see if the cat will use it. Every kitten is an individual and requires a separate solution for most problems. A toy or object from his former nest could be comforting to him. It would have a familiar odor on it that might offer some reassurance. Trial and error is the only way to find out. Some kittens are comforted by a softly playing radio turned to an all-night talk show. Soft music may work, too. It is a fact that young kittens will either cry all night or get into as much mischief as you allow. Of course they will sleep intermittently. A kitten that has been socialized properly at the earliest time will make the quickest adjustment to the new home. In any event, the worst will be over in a week or two. Some cats make an adjustment in one night, but don't count on it.

2

COOL CATS

There may be more cats in America than cars. It has been estimated that over 50 million American families own one or more of them, making cats the most popular pet of all. Of these, two or three million are purebred felines with predictable personalities. The point is that most house cats are not of any particular breed. How then, can one reasonably identify or define the personality of any one of them? And what about the personality of purebred cats?

If cats seem cool, it is because of the difficulty in defining their elusive personalities. There are, however, recognizable personality traits and characteristics that can be identified and assigned to each of the existing cat breeds. Of course, many of the breeds have similar or even identical personalities because they are simply variations of one another based on coat color and pattern. A number of cat breeds have been created by combining the characteristics of two or more existing breeds. Consequently, the personalities may represent a combination of traits from the various breeds involved while others may have formed a unique personality of their own.

What little knowledge there is of the feline personality comes from the scant scientific research that has been conducted and from the extensive experience of breeders, exhibitors, veterinarians, and knowledgeable pet owners. These are the people to ask for a more accurate description of the feline personality.

Feline personalities or temperaments are not as easily defined as the various canine temperaments. Because of the wide diversity of dog breeds and the extreme differences among them, each canine personality is sharply defined and more easily recognized. The differences in temperament among the dog breeds is much more obvious than among the cat breeds and is energetically displayed most of the time for all to see. The differences in feline personalities are subtle and known mostly to those fully experienced with one or more of the breeds. Cats do, indeed, have a mystery about them in their personal qualities and temperaments, which have seldom been classified in any particular manner.

To help the novice understand the pet he or she lives with, or for the person about to acquire a kitten, here is a concise description of the personalities of the various cat breeds. Also offered is a description of some general personality categories that apply to cats of mixed breed or unknown origin.

Admittedly, these personality categories have been arbitrarily created by the author and are not based on scientific inquiry. They are merely presented to the perplexed cat owner as a frame of reference for the purpose of comparison.

Purebred Cats

Purebred cats are like furry bonbons stepping out of chocolate boxes with red satin ribbons tied around their plush necks. With names like Scheherazade, Ashleigh, and Rapunzel, these felines of distinction have moved into the mainstream and are no longer beyond the reach of the average cat lover. In the recent past the elegance of a long-haired, white Persian or a sumptuous chocolate point Siamese could only be found in the luxurious homes of the rich and famous. Although purebred cats are expensive and require a bit of bother to find, they are definitely abundant and available to anyone who wants one.

The question that also seems to arise is whether a pure-bred cat is better than one that is not. The answer to that question depends on who you ask and what you mean by "better." A *generic* or mixed-breed cat usually costs far less money than a purebred cat (if it costs anything at all). Although most cats are either handsome, striking or beautiful, purebred cats are predictable in their look and personality and mixed-breed or *generic* cats are not. A properly bred Bombay kitten, for example, is definitely going to grow into an adult black cat that is gentle and quiet. How a mixed-breed kitten is going to turn out is anyone's guess. Still, one is not healthier than the other. Also, you cannot enter a mixed-breed or generic cat in a cat show for champion status.

Purebred cats, according to the largest and most impor-tant cat organization in the world, the Cat Fanciers' Asso-ciation, Inc. (CFA), " . . . can be divided into three types: *natu-ral, man-made,* and *spontaneous mutation.* Natural breeds such as the Persian, Russian Blue, Turkish Angora, and others were formed in nature's crucible, then stylized by cat fanciers through selective breeding. *Man-made* breeds—the Exotic Shorthair and Bombay, to name a few examples—were created by cat lovers who artfully combined existing breeds. *Spontaneous mutations* like the Manx and Scottish Fold are the consequence of nature's whimsical scrambling of the genetic code, which results in the taillessness in the Manx and the demurely capped ears in the [Scottish] Fold that are the respective signatures of these breeds."

The idea of maintaining specific cat breeds and keeping them pure is to preserve and possibly improve the ideal look and personality associated with the various breeds. The aesthetic beauty and temperament of any given breed can only be continued if someone understands and practices the science of genetics and selective breeding. Cats are carefully selected and bred for their best characteristics and eliminated from breeding programs for their faults. Individuals that do not measure up or are seriously flawed are usually rejected and not bred to other cats.

National cat associations such as the CFA adopt written standards for all the cat breeds accepted for registration by them. Individual cats of each breed are then judged in cat shows and compared to the standards of its breed. Cats that appear to be closer to representations of the standards of their breeds are declared winners and awarded a number of points toward earning a title such as Champion or Grand Champion. When purebred kittens are born the litter is registered with a registering organization. Each individual kitten is later registered by its owner with enough of its history so that a complete pedigree can be maintained on any registered cat. Many of those registered are then qualified to compete in cats shows around the country in an effort to win a title of Champion or Grand Champion.

The family history of any purebred cat is traceable, through its registered pedigree, which is filed with the registering association it belongs to. All purebred cats and their kittens must be registered with a national cat association if they are to authenticate their purebred status for other breeders and in order to qualify for cat shows. On the North American continent there are six national registering organizations that maintain files on purebred cats in addition to governing breed standards, sanctioning cat shows, and qualifying show judges. Among these organizations are the American Cat Association (ACA); the American Cat Fanciers' Association (ACFA); the Canadian Cat Association (CCA); the Cat Fanciers' Association (CFA); the Cat Fanciers' Federation (CFF); and The International Cat Association (TICA).

In the remainder of this chapter you will find a large section offering personality traits and some background information about each of the cat breeds that are accepted for registration by the various national cat associations. Following this is a brief section outlining the personality types that mixed-breed or generic cats might display. Whether you live with a purebred or generic cat this information is certain to help you understand your purr-fect friend.

Short Glossary

For the benefit of the inexperienced cat lover a short glossary of terms that are familiar to the cat breeder and exhibitor are offered here. These terms are used throughout the following breed personality section.

Agouti: pertaining to the hair color between the stripes of a tabby cat's coat pattern. The color is seen on each hair in a band. The color of the band is absent in solid colored cats.

Cobby: A body type—short-legged, sturdy, broad-chested, somewhat square in appearance. Persians are representative of this type.

Foreign: A body type—see **Svelte**.

Inbreeding: Breeding cats of the same family, such as a father to a daughter or a brother to a sister.

Mutation: A radical physical change in a cat from birth, which can lead to the creation of a new breed. The folded ears of the Scottish Fold is an important example.

Nose leather: Referring to the nasal skin and its subtle coloring.

Oriental: A body type—see Svelte.

Outcross: Mating unrelated cats of the same breed.

Peke-faced: The face resembling that of a Pekingese dog, with a very short, indented nose and wrinkled skin. A characteristic found in some Persians and long-haired mixed-breeds.

Points: The contrasting, darker colors on a cat's extremities, which include the mask (front of the face), bottom of the legs, tips of the ears, and the end of the tail. Seen in such breeds as the Siamese, Colorpoint Shorthair, Balinese, Javanese, and others.

Roman nose: A description of a nose type most commonly found on the Siamese and Rex. It is a nose that is characteristically high on the face with a prominent bridge.

Self: A cat's coat that is the same color all over as found on the Oriental Shorthair.

Svelte: A specific feline body type—long, slender and fine-boned, with a thin tapering tail and a long, tapering wedge-shaped head. Cats of this body type are sometimes referred to as "foreign." The Siamese is typical of this type as well as the many breeds developed from the Siamese.

Tabby: A complex coat color made up of the agouti background and an overlay of dark hair set in a striped pattern. The four types of tabby patterns are Classic, Mackerel, Spotted, and Ticked. Tabby coat patterns involve stripes on the body, rings on the tail, barring on the legs, lines (referred to as necklaces) on the neck, spots on the underside, and barring on the face with an *M*-shaped stripe on the forehead.

Tubular: A body type—see **Svelte**.

Type: The size and shape of a cat's body that are characteristic of a specific breed.

Personalities of the Breeds

Abyssinian

The personality of this breed is lively, energetic and quite active. Despite its sudden bursts of energy it is an even-tempered cat and quite pleasing to live with. It is an extremely curious cat and quite lively. Abyssinians are affectionate, playful cats that quickly win the hearts of their human families Allegedly, they descended from two small African wild cats and appear to represent the classical look of wild cats found in Abyssinia (Ethiopia) and/or Egypt, three or four thousand years ago. Some have written that they are descended from the ancient caffre cats or the sacred cats of Egypt. The breed first arrived in North America around the turn of the twentieth century.

Abyssinians are agile, solid and athletic-looking, and are enthusiastic about the things that interest them such as the four walls and the ceilings of their homes. They represent a beautiful balance of mind and body.

American Curl

American Curls are affectionate cats that love to sit on the shoulders of anyone who will let them. Adults are relaxed and playful and not as active as some of the Oriental breeds. They are agile, curious, and easily trained.

This is a recent breed accepted by the CFA for registration and showing. It was first recorded as a spontaneous mutation in Southern California. In order to be considered a bona fide American Curl a cat must be descended from "Shulamith," the foundation female from which all pedigreed American Curls descend. The distinguishing feature of the breed is the extraordinary formation of its ears. They stand erect, open, with an intriguing upward curve forming a moderate curl. The American Curl is now seen in both long-haired and short-haired coats.

American Shorthair

This breed's personality embodies the essence of the typical cat disposition. Many believe they represent the sum and substance of all cats, everywhere. They are self-assured individuals with strong egos and delightfully pleasing natures. They are, at times, high-spirited, playful, and very affectionate. American Shorthairs are also highly intelligent cats devoted to the business of hunting and all things connected with those labors. Although they possess sweet natures, they are independent, self-sufficient, and highly dignified creatures. The American Shorthair is a *working cat* with extraordinary hunting skills; it effortlessly detects the presence of rodents and captures them with great ease.

Although the breed is rooted to the basic working cats of Europe it is, nevertheless, an original purebreed native to the North American continent. Those who have painstakingly developed this remarkable breed over the decades bristle when it is confused with the generic, non-pedigreed, short-haired housecat that it seems to resemble. The mixed-breed housecat and the purebreed American Shorthair are very different cats. American Shorthairs have been selectively bred since 1904 with the best specimens chosen to be mated for their physical and mental excellence.

As a purebreed American Shorthairs differ from ordinary housecats because they have been bred for hundreds of generations to meet the high breed standards that keep them strong, muscular, intelligent, and lively. The breed's body has been developed over the decades for hard work with no aspect of its anatomy exaggerated, which could create weakness in its anatomy. The general goal is to create cats that are strongly built and well balanced, producing cats with power, endurance, and agility.

American Wirehair

The American Wirehair personality is most importantly a loving and sweet-natured one. Although they are more reserved than their American Shorthair cousins, they grow into loving, unassuming pets with friendly, bright personalities. At times you hardly know they are around.

Considered the result of a spontaneous mutation, the American Wirehair's origins can be traced to one cat, "Council Rock Farm Adam of Hi-Fi." With his sister, "Tip-Toe," he was born with fur that was springy, dense and resilient, resembling sheep wool. Considered a mutation of the American Shorthair, its coat distinguishes the breed from all the others. The hairs of the coat are either crimped, hooked, or bent, giving it a wiry appearance. These attention-getting cats have become an original American cat breed and have been bred to type with the help of the American Shorthair as its necessary outcross. They are wonderful companion animals for those who love a more subdued cat.

Balinese

The Balinese is a long-haired version of the Siamese with only a slight difference in personality. The difference has to do with intensity. These are slightly less vocal cats than their Siamese cousins with voices that are just a bit softer. Balinese are just as active as Siamese but have a less intense way of going about their business. They are a bit more easygoing and are perfect for those who love the look of the Siamese but not necessarily that much zest. The Balinese are warm, loving cats with enthusiasm and zeal. They do well with children.

The name Balinese is taken from the graceful dancers of Bali. They were first recognized as a separate breed in 1963 and have been produced consistently by knowledgeable breeders ever since. CFA allows them only in the four traditional color points of Siamese cats: seal point, chocolate point, blue point, and lilac point. *(Points are the contrasting, darker colors on a cat's extremities, which include the front of the face, bottom of the legs, tips of the ears, and the end of the tail.)* The Balinese is identical to another breed, the Javanese, which is another long-haired version of the Siamese but with sixteen color point varieties *(but not the four Siamese color points).* These are good-natured cats with an unquenchable curiosity. They insist on participating in all human activities and require a thorough combing and brushing on a daily basis. See *Javanese* and *Siamese* for more information.

Birman (Sacred Cat of Burma)

These large, long-haired cats are among the most striking-looking felines in the world and have personalities to match.

They are *color-pointed* cats, which means their coats are similar to those of the Siamese. Their bodies are seen in a pale, even color and their points (ears, legs, tail and mask) are seen in a darker, contrasting shade. The primary difference in coat color and pattern between the Birman and other color point breeds is the bottom inch or two of their legs, which are white. Their white tips are referred to in their standard as *gloves*.

Birmans are sometimes quiet and gentle and sometimes very active. They are highly intelligent cats and do not appreciate being left alone, which explains why they enjoy the company of their families so much. They thrive on the company of people, cats, and other pets and get along well with everyone including children. Birmans are easy to handle and are great companion animals.

Birmans were the temple cats of Lao-Tsun and were cared for and admired by the Buddhist priests. In Europe they have been referred to as the Tibetan Temple Cats. Because of a generous act of bravery, August Pavie and Major Russell-Gordon, both living in France, were given a pair of Birmans in 1919. The cats have been carefully nurtured in France since that time. They came to North America circa 1960.

The Birman is a *natural* breed and has no relationship to the Siamese despite its similar color point coat pattern. Its long hair and larger body type make it quite different. The white fur gloves at the end of all four paws help distinguish this breed from most others.

Bombay

The Bombay is a feline swatch of solid black velour with two copper-penny eyes staring softly out at the world. Gentle, mild-mannered and good-natured, these soft-spoken cats mix well with fellow cats, children and even with dogs.

Even though it resembles a friendly panther, the Bombay cannot bear to be left alone and craves the company of other living beings. These are charming, graceful felines. They are playful, soft-spoken and very affectionate.

The first Bombay was the result of a mating between a Burmese and a black American Shorthair in the United States. The breed was created in 1958 but was not accepted for championship showing by the Cat Fanciers' Association until 1976. It was named for the black leopards of India.

The ideal Bombay is a unique-looking cat with a short, deep black coat that glistens to a shine. Its eyes are usually copper-colored but are gold in some. It is not simply a "black cat" that you walk around on the street. This breed with its solid, muscular body is far from an ordinary-looking cat. The sweet expression on its face, its alert, friendly manner and its surprising weight for its size make it an outstanding purebred cat.

British Shorthair

Although it is no longer practiced, there was a period after World War I when English breeders outcrossed the British Shorthair with Persians to create a larger, more massive-looking short-haired cat. This, of course, explains the difference in size between the American Shorthair, which is somewhat smaller, and the British Shorthair. It also has a bearing on the personality differences between the two breeds. The British Shorthair is a more docile cat than the American Shorthair and is calm, quiet and peaceful which is similar to the Persian personality.

Although British Shorthairs are not very playful beyond kittenhood they are not aloof but, rather, are friendly, reserved cats. The most striking aspect of this breed's personality is its gentleness, despite its great sense of dignity.

The British Shorthair was accepted in the United States for registration and showing in the 1970s. Ideal examples of the breed show a compact, powerful body with a large, deep chest. Despite its short to medium legs it appears to stand taller than its American cousin. Its most outstanding physical feature is its massive head, which is round and wide, well set on a short, thick neck. Its cheeks are full and round. The coat is short and very dense. This breed is slow to mature and, surprisingly, has a faint voice that is hard to hear when beyond earshot. It is important to understand that the British Shorthair is distinctly different in many ways from the American Shorthair.

Burmese

Here is yet another breed with a fabulous, outgoing personality, which contradicts the misconception that cats are aloof, independent and self-possessed. The Burmese is an exceptionally friendly breed, especially with children, and enjoy curling up in bed with anyone who will allow them this luxury. They are soft-spoken, yet active cats with engaging personalities. Burmese are highly intelligent animals that crave the love and warmth of their families. They love to be with people and dislike being alone. In that sense, their personalities resemble the Siamese who love to interact directly with the humans they live with. Burmese live happier in pairs, especially when all members of the family are gone during the day.

The first Burmese in America was a brown female Oriental-type cat named Wong Mau who was the mother of the entire American Burmese breed. Resembling a dark-colored Siamese, Wong Mau arrived in the United States in 1930 and was mated with a Siamese for lack of another Burmese. Because the cat originated in Rangoon its owner Dr. Joseph G. Thompson of San Francisco called his new breed *Burmese. The Cat-Book Poems*, dating from the Ayudhya period of Siam (1350–1767), picture the Burmese on a page with the Siamese, the Korat, and a black cat with a white collar called the Singha-sep. All the descendants of this historic line of great cats have a sumptuous dark brown or Sable coat color. At one time the Cat Fanciers' Association only accepted the Burmese in Sable (a rich, dark brown). It now registers the Burmese in Champagne (honey-colored beige), Blue (soft, warm bluish-gray), and Platinum (silvery-gray with pale-fawn undertones). Other cat associations register Burmese in colors other than Sable as a separate breed called the Malayan.

Chartreux

The Chartreux are large, working cats who are excellent at keeping the rodent population in check. They are amiable, friendly cats with just about any human, especially with members of their families. Although they are quite tolerant of visitors and other cats they do not thrive best in a busy, noisy household. They resemble the British Shorthair ("British Blue") in dimensions, look and personality.

A native of France, this ancient breed is the center of many heated discussions in the Cat Fancies of Europe where some argue it is simply the French version of the English breed, the British ("Blue") Shorthair. The origins of the Chartreux are commonly thought to be from the monks of the Carthusian monastery, La Grand Chartreuse, near Grenoble, France, where the liqueur Chartreuse was created.

These brawny French cats are valued for their hunting prowess and robust look, not the least of which includes their dense, water-repellent haircoat. Though powerfully built, Chartreux are extremely limber cats that can jump gracefully with the rest of catkind. There are no traces of coarseness or clumsiness in this breed. They are, in fact, quite refined. Males are slower to mature than females but grow to be much larger. A true representation of the Chartreux breed is strong, intelligent, independent, yet affectionate and very adaptive.

Colorpoint Shorthair

It cannot be denied that almost all personality traits of this breed are similar to the Siamese. Colorpoint Shorthair characteristics are keen intelligence, liveliness, vocalness, and extreme affection. At times their behavior is somewhat canine in their desire to fetch, stand on their back legs, beg, and do some of the tricks associated with dogs. They constantly "talk" and follow members of the family wherever they go.

Colorpoint Shorthairs for all intents and purposes are Siamese cats with all the same coat and point patterns as the Siamese but are not allowed to have the traditional Siamese point colors (i.e., seal point, chocolate point, blue point, and lilac point) by the Cat Fanciers' Association. *(Points are the contrasting, darker colors on a cat's extremities, which include the front of the face, bottom of the legs, tips of the ears, and the end of the tail.)*

The CFA accepts the following Colorpoint Shorthair colors: Red Point, Cream Point, Seal Lynx Point, Chocolate Lynx Point, Blue Lynx Point, Lilac Lynx Point, Red Lynx Point, Seal-Tortie Point, Chocolate-Tortie Point, Blue-Cream Point, Lilac-Cream Point, Seal-Tortie Lynx Point, Chocolate-Tortie Lynx Point, Blue-Cream Lynx Point, Lilac-Cream Lynx Point, and Cream Lynx Point.

The Colorpoint Shorthair is registered as a separate breed by CFA, partly because traditional Siamese breeders do not wish to permit any but the four traditional color points and partly because the breed was crossed with American Shorthairs to introduce the new colors. Siamese breeders argue that this means they are not pure Siamese cats. Complicating the issue further is the Oriental Shorthair, which is another nontraditional version of the Siamese. It does not have color points on the extremities of its body, but rather, shows a solid color over the entire body.

Like the Siamese, they are of average cat-size, polished-looking, lean with long ebbing lines, and have very supple but muscular bodies. Males are usually larger.

Cornish Rex

The personality of the Cornish Rex and its close relative, the Devon Rex, is quite similar to the Siamese. This is an intensely curious, affectionate, needful breed that requires the care and affection of its human family. Like the Siamese, they are highly talkative and delightfully communicative. They are very playful as kittens once they adjust to their new surroundings.

Like the Devon Rex, the Cornish Rex is most noticed for its part wavy, part curly undercoat which is sparsely distributed over its long and elegant, slender body. The unusual haircoat has no topcoat which tends to exaggerate the ears and facial features, making them look larger than they are. The Rex has a profoundly different look from other breeds that is perfect for the cat lover with a desire for the unusual. The breed is unmistakable. These are small-to-medium cats with lean bodies and wavy haircoats.

The Cornish Rex came about by spontaneous mutation

in a litter of kittens born to a white domestic shorthair on a farm in Cornwall, England, in 1950. When the kitten, named Kallibunker, matured, he was mated back to his mother, a short-haired cat with straight hair. The Rex was created as a breed when several of Kallibunker's kittens were born with curly coats. The name Rex was given to the breed after the popular curly coated rabbit type. There are two separate recessive genes that cause the curly coat: Gene I (the Cornish) and Gene II (the Devon). Because the Devon cannot be mated to the Cornish and produce the curly coat they have been established as two separate breeds.

The Cornish Rex is an affectionate cat and, it is said, will wag its tail when happy, just like a dog. Both Rex breeds have garnered great public attention at cat shows because of their striking coats which resemble the "Marcel Wave," a famous women's hairstyle of the 1930s. Rex cats are heavier than they look and are pleasant to touch. Their bodies are not as angular as they appear and are actually gently curved. Members of this breed are smart, aware of what is happening around them, and generally pleasant to hold.

Cymric

The Cymric personality is identical to the personality of the Manx because this breed is essentially a tailless Manx with long hair. Like their short-haired cousin, the Manx, Cymrics are happy, friendly, and loving with some humans, but not with others. They are gentle and quiet—until it is time to hunt. They are competent predators and always surprise their families with the ruthlessness of their hunting skills.

Until recent times, the CFA simply regarded the Cymric as a long-haired Manx. It is now registered and shown as a separate breed with all the privileges accorded any registerable breed. Because long-haired kittens have appeared in Manx litters for years the Cymric is not considered a hybrid (man-made breed). All Manx parents must have the long-hair gene to produce Cymric kittens. Definition of Cymric is *of the Welsh*.

The tailless Cymric has a rounded head with prominent cheeks. It is a broad-chested cat with thick, short front legs and longer hind legs giving it a rabbitlike hop when it runs. The haircoat consists of a thick, double coat of medium length with an attractive gloss shining from its surface. Like the short-coated Manx it is a sweet-natured animal that always stays alert and curious. They are surprisingly heavy when lifted. Cymrics do not mature as quickly as other breeds.

Devon Rex

Although the Devon Rex resembles the Cornish Rex, especially with its unusually wavy coat, it is a separate breed. Without exception, all cat associations treat these two breeds separately because of their genetic differences. The Devon Rex was discovered ten years after the Cornish Rex in Devon, England.

Although the Devon Rex has a somewhat Siamese look its personality is different. As a matter of fact, some believe there are slight personality differences between the Devon and the Cornish Rex breeds. The Devon is somewhat less talkative than the Cornish and much less talkative than the Siamese. The two Rex breeds are calm, quiet lap cats— gently playful with outstanding personalities. Both breeds are readily identified by their part wavy, part curly coats, by their slender, supple bodies, their wedged-shaped heads, wide, slightly oval-shaped eyes, and lengthy, Roman nose.

Egyptian Mau

Egyptian Maus are friendly cats with their families but are also very active, indoors and out. This can present a problem for the wise cat lover who does not allow his or her pet to roam freely. Taking them out for walks while attached to a leash and harness is a workable solution. It allows them to get the exercise they need, but at the same time prevents them from getting into trouble. Some owners have constructed large, outdoor pens for this breed. These are people-loving cats and they cannot tolerate being shut away for long periods of time. The alternative is to simply accept the high activity level of the breed and learn to enjoy the sometimes frenzied running about Egyptian Maus indulge in.

These are uncommon cats with their cheetahlike spotted coat and their gooseberry-green eyes which can turn to an amber color with emotional disturbance. They have been officially accepted for showing and registering by the CFA since the late 1970s but are not seen in many homes as pets. This is due in part to their high cost and in part to their reserved personalities which vary between aloofness and sociability.

These cats do not warm up well to strangers despite the fact that they are very affectionate with members of their own families. Their greatest appeal involves living with an animal that reminds us of the wildness from which all cats come. The Mau possesses that most typical catlike quality of aloof reserve with strangers while allowing only a few close relationships.

This is a natural breed that seems to be halfway between the Oriental and cobby look. It strikes a delicate balance between the compactness of a Burmese and the slim elegance of the Siamese. The coat pattern and colors of the Mau are its most distinctive features with random spots dotted over a silver, bronze, or smoke ground color. The Mau's eyes are bright gooseberry green. The breed is moderately vocal but almost sings when handled. Their voices are soft and mellow. Egyptian Maus are one-of-a-kind cats.

Exotic Shorthair

These are heavyset swains that are loving pets with sweet dispositions and are said to get along with children quite well. Depending on the quality of their breeding and early handling they range in disposition from total friendliness with everyone to cool reserve with strangers. Most enjoy a lot of fuss and handling while some barely tolerate any attention at all. A few bristle at the slightest handling such as combing and brushing. These intelligent cats are good at keeping the rodent population under control. Although they are sweet-natured, affectionate, and gentle, they are often seriously reflective as they settle into one comfortable position to think things over.

The Exotic Shorthair is a hybrid or man-made breed and was created by crossing Persians with American Shorthairs. The idea was to achieve the medium-to-large cobby build and massive, round head of the Persian with the medium-length, thick coat of the American Shorthair. The result has been something like a short-haired Persian. This interesting breed has been recognized by the CFA since 1966.

It is a successful hybridization resulting in sweet, gentle cats that are easy-to-groom Persians. Exotic Shorthairs like a good romp once in a while but do not seem to be destructive. They are good with other cats and are even-tempered.

They are ideal pets offering the massive Persian look and with low-maintenance coats.

Havana Brown

These are lively, very playful cats that are intelligent and agile, making them diabolically clever in the trouble they can get into. The personality of the Havana Brown is profoundly influenced by the two breeds that were crossed to create this breed. This breed is the result of crossing a Siamese with a Domestic Shorthair (in England). From its Siamese background the Havana is a cat that interacts greatly with people. From its Domestic Shorthair background it is a hardy cat that loves to hunt. These are sweet and loving cats, with personalities that combine a rich blend of intelligence and devotion.

Havana Browns are easy to groom and make great family companions. They are good-natured and affectionate, good with children, somewhat trainable, and not as vocal as the Siamese.

They were bred in the 1950s from Siamese, Russian Blues, and black domestic shorthairs to achieve their beautiful brown coats and Siamese body types. These bright, active cats resemble the Burmese. Their coats are dark mahogany-toned brown resembling cured tobacco deep down to the roots of each hair. Even their whiskers are brown.

Japanese Bobtail

Japanese Bobtails always seem to be busy running from one place to another. They are family-oriented and quite devoted to their families whether they are humans, cats, or cats and humans together. They seem to relate to each other quite well. These are highly intelligent creatures with friendly, personal warmth and charm that makes them ideal housecats. Bobtails are an uncommon breed, and not seen in too many homes outside of Japan. They are affectionate, playful, inquisitive and somewhat assertive as they have a tendency to dominate many human situations.

They are usually serious cats that become playful only on occasion. The Japanese Bobtail has been seen on the streets of Japan for centuries as well as in many homes and temples there. The breed has been recorded in the Japanese art and culture for as long as they have been in Japan.

The tricolors are preferred the most in Japan because they are thought to bring good luck. The Japanese call them Mi-Ki. In the United States the red, black and white calico pattern is thought to be the most pleasing. These cats can be recognized by their charming personalities, their somewhat slanted eyes, and, of course, by their bobbed tails, which can be any shape imaginable. Their short tails should resemble that of a bunny tail with the hair fanning out to create a pom-pom appearance which effectively camouflages the underlying bone structure of the tail.

Javanese

In order to understand the personality of this breed it is important to know that the Javanese is simply a Siamese with long hair (like the Balinese) but with sixteen allowable varieties of color points. *(Points are the contrasting, darker colors on a cat's extremities, which include the front of the face, bottom of the legs, tips of the ears, and the end of the tail.)* The Siamese (and the Balinese) are only allowed four different color points *(seal point, chocolate point, blue point, lilac point)*. The Cat Fanciers' Association

(CFA) registers the Javanese as a separate breed because it is allowed many different color point coats (but not the four Siamese color points). This means that the Javanese (and the Balinese) is almost the same cat as the Siamese but with different color points in addition to long hair. Therefore, its personality is identical in most respects to Siamese cats.

Some fanciers believe that the only personality difference between the Javanese and the Siamese has to do with intensity. The voices of Javanese cats are a bit softer than that of their Siamese cousins and they are slightly less vocal. They are not quite as noisy as the Siamese and have a less intense way of going about their business. The Javanese are ideal cats for those who enjoy the beautiful look and personality of the Siamese but with just a bit less exuberance. They are lively, demanding, affectionate, and very nice for children.

They can be very demanding and they do it with incessant vocalizing. They are good-natured cats with an unquenchable curiosity, insisting on participating in all human activities. See *Balinese* and *Siamese* for more information.

Korat

The personality of the Korat can be characterized by its quiet energy. Although it is well-suited to family life it does not thrive in a household with boistrous or highly energized children. These are smart cats that are good with other animals but are essentially quiet, soft-spoken and responsive to human handling. Those that were originally brought over from England were possessed of a sweeter personality than those that were bred in the United States. In the United States it is best to acquire individuals from breeders that select for sweet, gentle temperament rather than for conformation.

The Korat is a playful friend and is responsive to human attention. Strong bonds develop quickly with these aesthetically pleasing animals. They are allowed only one coat color by CFA and that is silver-blue all over, tipped with silver which is supposed to produce a halo effect.

Native to the ancient Province of Korat in Thailand (now known as Nakhon Ratchasima), they are a natural breed often called by their native Thai names, Si-Sawat, which means, "a cat with the color of the Look-Sawat," a wild fruit plant whose seed is a silver-blue color. This ancient breed was described and pictured in *The Cat-Book Poems* (circa 18th century), and now in the Bangkok National Museum. The Korat is one of the oldest recorded breeds in history. It was recognized by the Cat Fanciers' Association in 1966.

This rare breed is more frequently seen in the United, States than in its native Thailand, its country of origin because of its secured place in the world of cat shows. Still, it is admired by the Thai people because of its image as a "good luck" cat.

Maine Coon Cat

The dominant features of the Maine Coon personality are confidence, self-assurance, and boldness. They are extremely likable cats with a casual, breezy manner. They are assertive in their style of play, despite their weak voices. The Maine Coon adjusts to other cats, and even dogs, with ease and comfort, but tends to dominate most situations. They are formidable hunters. Mice, beware.

Maine Coon Cats are a true native American breed, first seen in the Northeastern part of the United States without benefit of a formal breeding program. These shaggy beauties were always prized as working cats as well as companion animals in the New England region, the place of their origin. It took many decades before they became a fully recognized breed, transforming from a farm worker and backyard cat to a CFA competitor. They did not become eligible for championship showing in the CFA until 1976. These are outgoing, lovable cats and almost totally self-sufficient, if their situation demands it. Despite their appearance, they are not the result of a mating between a cat and a raccoon.

The brown tabby varieties have rings on their big bushy tails like raccoon's. The Maine Coon Cat, a natural breed, has come to be accepted as an indigenous American cat. Prized by New Englanders as being the largest, smartest and most beautiful cat anywhere, the amiable Maine Coon Cat is thought to be the by-product of short-haired, domestic cats, brought to the United States by the Pilgrims in 1640, and Angora cats, brought by seafaring New Englanders to these shores in the 1800s.

Originally a working cat, the solid, rugged Maine Coon Cat can endure harsh climates. A distinctive characteristic is its smooth, shaggy coat. With an essentially amiable disposition, it has adapted to varied environments.

Manx

The Manx personality exudes a charming form of mischief that makes it difficult to express anger at them. They are bright, energetic, vivacious creatures with highly lovable ways about them. Although they are not difficult to train they do require discipline from time to time to prevent their robust behavior from becoming troublesome. Their distinctive personalities are borne out of their great intelligence. These are playful but stubborn cats. Give them empty boxes, bags, or bowls and they will play away their energy.

Originating from the Isle of Man in the Irish Sea, Manx are different from most other shorthair breeds because they have no tails. Actually, they are seen in three types of tails: the *rumpy*, no tail at all; the *stumpy*, a tail stump of one to five inches; or the *longie*, the presence of a complete tail. Only the tailless Manx, however, is accepted for show. The tailed cats are important because when *rumpies* are bred together for three generations the kittens do not survive.

The Manx are friendly, outgoing cats with everyone and are quite capable of suddenly jumping on the lap or even the shoulder of a visitor in your house, if they are so inclined. They are also superb hunters, catching mice (and other prey animals) with great ease. Manx are medium-sized, robust cats with high hind quarters. Their back legs are much longer than their forelegs causing the rump to be higher than the shoulders. When they run they resemble rabbits hopping in the grass. Despite the fact that these are short-haired cats they have plush, double coats that are thick and abundant.

Norwegian Forest Cat

Norwegian Forest Cats are independent animals that enjoy the outdoors. These robust cats love to climb trees and are extremely playful, intelligent and affectionate. They prefer open spaces and are best suited for country living where they are excellent hunters. Although they accept domestic life and like human company they are cautious with strangers and prefer living in houses that offer them a certain amount of freedom.

Despite the similarity in appearance to the Maine Coon

Cat, the Norwegian Forest Cat is a separate breed. Its back legs are longer than the front legs so that its rump is higher than its shoulders. This clearly distinguishes it from the Maine Coon Cat.

References to the "Norsk Skogkatt" have appeared in Scandinavian poetry, legends, and writings for hundreds of years. It was recognized and shown in Oslo long before World War II, but has only recently been accepted in the CFA.

These are very slow-maturing cats, not reaching their full growth until approximately five years of age. At about eight to twelve months of age the development of the skull may cause the eyes to appear too round; this can be forgiven in the show ring at that time, but not much beyond that age.

Ocicat

Even though the Ocicat resembles a ferocious leopard or ocelot it is pure pussycat. These are friendly, even-tempered cats that become totally devoted to the people in their lives. In keeping with their appearance, they are not timid cats and do not run and hide when visitors come calling. On the contrary, they are quite confident and somewhat extraverted not matter who is in the house. Nevertheless, Ocicats are neither wild nor dangerous. They are friendly and gentle like all domesticated cats.

Their spotted coats suggest a similarity to the ocelot, which is a wild, spotted leopardlike cat, native to the southwestern United States. These hybrids were created by the interbreeding of Siamese, Abyssinian, and American Shorthairs. They are attention-getting cats that draw a large crowd at cat shows. Their outgoing personalities reflect their Abyssinian-Siamese genes.

Oriental Shorthair

There are few differences in personality between Oriental Shorthairs and Siamese. The primary difference between the two breeds has to do with the color patterns of their coats. The Siamese has color points (restricted to seal point, chocolate point, blue point, lilac point) and the Oriental Shorthair has a *self* or solid color or patterned coat.

Oriental Shorthairs, like the Siamese, are magnificent companion animals for those who desire a cat that will talk to them and follow them everywhere. They are quite intelligent creatures with a unique charm all their own that possibly comes from a self-assurance bordering on arrogance. Everything they do is done with grace, wit, and elegance and watching them can be quite entertaining as though attending a show.

However, these are active, high-jumping cats capable of great mischief. Many are clever with their paws and capable of opening cupboards, refrigerator doors and some drawers. They can be highly assertive, vocal cats once they decide they want something specific from you. When they get in their assertion mode it is usually for food, or your absolute, undivided attention.

According to the CFA the breed evolved "from the basic Siamese/domestic shorthair/Abyssinian hybrid crosses . . ." The Siamese gave it type (and personality) and the domestic shorthair gave it color. The standards for the Oriental Shorthair and the Siamese are almost identical except for color and coat pattern. The ideal Oriental Shorthair is a svelte cat with long, tapering lines, very lithe but muscular.

Persian

Among the purebreeds, Persians are the most popular,

most prolific, and most admired of all cats. More Persians are entered in all-breed cat shows than any other breed. Persian cats are spectacular-looking with their long, puffy coats and haughty facial expressions that seem to convey benign distain. They tend to command a great deal of attention in the show ring as well as in the front parlor. Although their physical beauty is more of the obvious kind than in other breeds their personalities come as a surprise to those who do not know them.

Persians are not very active, to say the least. These are cats that are best suited to those who would like a serene companion that is capable of sitting quietly for hours, staring out at a world that does not particularly impress them. Much of their day and night is spent sleeping. They eat, move about a bit, rub up against a family member for food, and then go back to their silent, social criticism.

Persians do have a beautiful sound when they deign to meow and they are considered to be well-behaved and good-mannered. They enjoy some attention but usually from one, perhaps two, members of their immediate family. These long-haired beauties have an aristocratic air about them but are affectionate, sociable (at times), and playful at home. Some of them even chase mice. They are among the most beautiful cats in the world and they exude great dignity. Few breeds are as popular or as successful.

There is nothing dainty about Persians. Under all that fluffy coat, is a stocky, heavy body supported by legs that are short, thick, and strong.

Ragdoll

These are gentle, docile cats that are not terribly active unless stimulated by play. Little seems to upset them except a late dinner. They enjoy the company of humans and particularly like to be held. It is said that the name of their breed came from the limp position they go into when held like a baby. They have pleasant personalities and are sweet to live with, talk to, and generally hang out with. They like people and enjoy the fuss and attention usually given despite the fact that their responses are not terribly energized. They require a safe and secure home.

Ragdolls are large cats, males weighing between fifteen and twenty pounds, females weighing between nine and twelve pounds. They are still uncommon and require a bit of effort and research to acquire.

Russian Blue

The Russian Blue temperament can be characterized as quiet, gentle, and affectionate. Although these are sweetly shy cats they are well-disposed toward children and other pets. They are often restrained and somewhat noncommittal when approached by those they do not know. Russian Blues are fine companion cats and become quite attached to their families. They seem to prefer an indoor life and that makes them perfect for city living. These gentle Russians have a very soft, quiet voice which is either an advantage or a disadvantage, depending on your likes and dislikes.

The most striking feature of this breed is its plush, dense coat which is short and easy to groom and similar to that of a beaver or a seal. In the parlance of the Cat Fancy, a *blue coat* indicates a rich blue-gray color. In the case of the Russian Blue, the double coat of this warm, sumptuous-looking cat is *blue* with outer guard hairs tipped with silver creating a glistening effect. The lavender-pink color of the paw pads and their vivid green eyes add to their exquisite beauty.

Scottish Fold

Sweet serenity characterizes the even temperament of this highly unusual breed. They not only have a unique appearance, due to their unusual ear structure, but they are so calm and laid back that one would hardly be aware of their presence if it wasn't for their conspicuous presence. Scottish Folds crave human companionship and are ideal pets for those who do not want a highly spirited animal tearing around the house. They are good-natured, warm, and exceptionally friendly. Even though they are hardy cats, like their domestic short-hair ancestors, they have very small voices and hardly ever use them. These strong, silent types are quite likely to stay in one resting place for hours without moving an inch. Those who live with Scottish Folds become so enamored of them they give them anything they want.

These cats are called the Scottish Fold because of their unique ears, the top halves of which fold forward, giving them an unusual look. The breed was created from a mutation of an unusual recessive gene that causes the ears to fold down in the middle. The kittens are born with straight ears. If the ears are going to fold over it happens in about three to four weeks. Only folded ear cats of Scottish lineage are permitted in the show ring. However, the straight-ear kittens are important for breeding purposes. Other outstanding features are their eyes. They are like large drops of sweet syrup that stare out at you with affection.

Siamese

One never truly owns the Siamese but, rather, has a relationship with it. The Siamese personality is highly complex because of their keen intelligence and fluctuating emotions. These cats seem to be exuberant and devoted one day and obstinate and sullen the next. Some have likened them to dogs in their desire to retrieve, do tricks and relate to their human families. They are, rather, more like humans in their desire to relate to their people in a highly vocal manner. They "talk" and "talk" and "talk." They follow specific family members around when they want something and it isn't always food.

Siamese cats are smart, affectionate and very, very pleasing friends to have in one's life. They stick their noses in everyone's business; jump into laps when people least expect it; and are very demanding of your attention. They will become very assertive and demanding if you attempt to read, write a letter, or talk on the telephone without looking at them or petting them. The minds of Siamese cats approach feline genius. They are intelligent animals with an affectionate nature and a strong desire to be a lively, active member of the family they live with.

Siamese cats are a natural, ancient breed, and are looked upon as a regal animal by those that live with them. They are often used for cross-breeding in serious breeding programs for their svelte type or magnificent color points. Many of today's unusual and popular breeds such as the Havana Brown, Himalayan, and Tonkinese are the result of these cross-breeding experiments. The outstanding physical feature of these beautiful cats is their contrasting color pattern referred to as *color points. (The term points refers to the darker facial mask, ears, legs, and tail which are seen in a lighter color that is in contrast to the rest of the body.)* In North America, only the four traditional color points are considered Siamese. They are seal point, chocolate point, blue point, and lilac point.

There are a number of svelte-type breeds that are varieties

of the traditional Siamese. The Balinese is a long-haired version that is seen in the four traditional color points. The Javanese is another long-haired version of the Siamese but seen in many other color points but not in the four traditional colors. The Colorpoint Shorthair is considered by many to be a Siamese but seen in a wide variety of color points other than the four traditional colors. And then there is the Oriental Shorthair, which is considered to be a Siamese but seen only in solid or tabby patterned colors.

Singapura

These are quiet, loving cats with an insatiable curiosity about everything connected with their families and their families' possessions. They are outgoing companion animals with a special talent for picking up on the various moods of the people they live with and relating to them in a special way. Singapuras are playful, active, sociable, and extremely maternal with people as well as kittens. These are "people" cats and develop strong attachments to their families.

The Singapura is a natural breed originating in Southeast Asia, particularly on the island nation of Singapore, at the south end of the Malay Peninsula, from which these cats take their name. The breed was common to the streets of Singapore and was seen and admired there by several Americans who imported them to the United States in 1975. An additional import entered the U.S. in 1980. The Singapura was accepted by the CFA for chamionship competition in 1988. They are small cats with a ticked coat pattern similar to that of the Abyssinian. Both breeds resemble miniature cougars. All other characteristics of the Singapura are different from those of the Abyssinian. Its coat, with its reddish-brown color and two bands of dark ticking separated by light bands, makes it a very attractive cat.

Somali

The Somali personality is similar to that of the Abyssinian with its high energy activity and inclinations for speedy runs across your house. Lively, intelligent, and shrew, Somalis are vigorous house cats that express their affection freely. And, they are fun-loving creatures. Give them a fluttering peacock feather, a bouncing Ping-Pong ball, or an empty shopping bag and they will give you a show that is almost as entertaining as when they run vertically up your wall.

Somalis and Abyssinians are almost identical cats except for the length of their coats. Somalis began as long-haired mutations of the Abyssinian. They have a fine, double coat that is of medium length with a full brush tail giving them an outstanding look, and placing them in the longhair category.

Admired for their similar appearance to the fox, their coats retain all the characteristic Abyssinian features, such as the agouti coloring (each hair is individually striped with brown or black) and the four Abyssinian colors: blue, ruddy, red, and fawn.

Tonkinese

Tonkinese love people. They are bold cats that are not even afraid of strangers in your home or outdoor traffic and noises. They are friendly, affectionate pets, and exceptionally good with children. These are cats with fun-loving personalities but at the same time can be full of mischief. They are playful—too playful for some. Because of the curious aspect of their personalities they will take outdoor walks with you and readily accept a leash and harness. In some respects, they have many of the Siamese behavioral traits.

Tonkinese are hybrids resulting from matings with the Siamese and the Burmese. The differences between the two contributing breeds have to do with the shape of their bodies and the color of their coats. Their bodies show a balance between the svelte type (slender, tubular-shaped, fine-boned) and the cobby type (deep-chested, large-boned, compact). Unlike the Siamese, the Tonkinese's point color does not contrast sharply with its ground coat color. The body color is always seen in a dilution (lighter shade) of the same, darker point color. CFA allows the Tonkinese coat to appear in four colors: natural mink, Champagne mink, blued mink, and platinum mink.

Turkish Angora

This is a gorgeous cat wrapped in a long, silky-soft, white fur coat (pure white is the most popular color). It is the personification of the feline presence and, for some, is the most beautiful of all the cat breeds. Owners tend to name them Harlow, Marilyn, Madonna.

The Turkish Angora is fastidiously clean and is a gentle, curious animal. It is a playful cat and is said to be responsive to training if given a lot of attention. It is quite sociable with its family, but thinks of itself as the leading player in its own home. These are cats with star quality. It does not like to share the spotlight with other cats. The Turkish Angora is not at all talkative. It is an intelligent and affectionate animal that is alert and, at times, quite lively. This cat likes what all cats like—close contact and good food.

Ankara (Angora), Turkey, is the birthplace of this luxurious-looking feline. The original Angoras were near extinction in the early twentieth century, and were being supplanted by those that were crossed with Persians. They are among the oldest longhair breeds and have been long admired in Turkey, their homeland.

Thanks to the Ankara zoo, the breed was rescued from extinction and carefully preserved in its true, ancient type. It was at the Ankara zoo where it was discovered in 1962. Two pairs were brought to North America and then established as the breed we know today. It was accepted for registration by the CFA in 1970 and advanced to championship status in 1973.

Mixed-breed Cats

The majority of house cats kept as pets are mixed-breeds. They are the result of random matings of various cat breeds or other mixed-breed cats. They are usually not registered, have no pedigree (record of ancestors), and are not considered to be purebred cats. The millions upon millions of people who own and live with such cats have no interest in these matters. In the United States they may be referred to as *house cats* or *alley cats*. In Great Britain they are sometimes called *moggs*.

The Cat Fancy has gone to great lengths to acknowledge the desirability of *all* cats by allowing household pets to be registered (by some cat associations) and by encouraging a household pet competition for ribbons and prizes in most cat shows. To qualify for one of these competitions all cats (not kittens) must be neutered; must have all of their physical properties (except for a tail in the case of Manx types); and may not be declawed. Unlike purebred cats, they are not judged according to a written standard but on the basis of physical condition, cleanliness, presentation, temperament, and attractive or unusual appearance.

Throughout the world, cats of unknown lineage comprise the vast majority of house pets and most of them are mixed-breeds. They are, without a doubt, the most popular cats of all.

Personalities of the Mixed-breeds

Lincoln *should* have said, "God must have loved the common cat, he made so many of them."

One of the most interesting aspects of cat ownership is personality type. Believing that all cats are alike is a misconception. They are not. The differences may seem obscure to those who have not been exposed to a wide variety of cats, but feline personalities are clearly distinct and well delineated to the experienced cat person. One need only read the previous section, "Personalities of the Breeds," to know just how different one breed is from another. However, we are at a disadvantage when trying to predict a cat's personality type without knowing its breed characteristics or its parents. What may help is the establishment of general personality categories for all cats, both purebred and mixed-breed.

Although all wild and domestic cats share a common set of behaviors and instincts (see Chapter Three, "Cat Scan"), there are a number of behavioral *styles* in which various cats express instinctive actions and responses. These so-called styles are what we commonly refer to as *temperament* or *personality*. They can easily be classified into several personality categories and are offered here to all cat fanciers. It is quite likely that a cat will possess more than one of the following personality traits. Even so, there is always one aspect of a cat's personality that is more pronounced than all the others and that is the one that should determine any given cat's personality category.

Assertive

Cats with assertive personalities are characterized by their lack of self-doubt. It never occurs to such cats that you might actually say no to them about anything. They insist on waking you out of a sound sleep in the morning so that you can feed them, and will not accept the idea of a closed door when they want to see various members of their family.

Assertive cats are usually very playful and will do everything in their power to get people to indulge their spirited moods. They are quite manipulative. Such cats are almost always frisky, except when they are napping. They will respond to the slightest attention given them. Cats that are assertive are highly intelligent and are usually quite charming because they assume everyone loves them. Most assertive cats are not afraid of people or new situations. Among those breeds that represent this personality category are the American Shorthair, Malayan, Manx, and Maine Coon Cat.

Sedate

The sedate cat is almost always calm and laid back. It is not lazy. It is not bored. It is not even tired. It is simply a creature that is at peace with its environment and usually too large a cat to go running around. Such cats enjoy the attention they receive from humans that live with them but only acknowledge this on a limited basis. They do not wish to spoil them. Sedate cats allow the world to come to them, bringing affectionate offerings of things that taste good and a great deal of attention.

Sedate cats are always pampered and accept the attention paid to them in a reserved, tolerant manner but always with just an edge of disdain. Although they do move around, from the food bowl to the litter pan, they slowly but constantly pursue with great success their life's work, which is to get as much rest as possible. Some sedate cats have a regal, aloof air about them, while others appear to be too spent to care one way or the other. Sedate cats are always grateful to be allowed to sleep, nap, or just sit quietly and think. Breeds typical of the sedate personality are the Persian, Scottish Fold, and Ragdoll.

Energetic

You can always recognize the home of a cat with an energetic personality by the paw prints that go up the wall and across the ceiling and down the opposite wall. Energetic cats pace about like restless tigers in a zoo cage and then suddenly race across the room like a Harley Davidson on open road.

The owners of such cats usually have snagged threads and tiny claw marks on their clothing due to the leaps their pets make onto them, suddenly and without warning. High-energy cats are easily distracted, excitable, and responsive to the slightest attention given to them, unless they are investigating an unfamiliar sound or movement. They usually know their name and come running at the sound of it, or at least turn and look. Energetic cats are rarely afraid of anything, are usually quite friendly, and move like lightning. Most of them are highly trainable. Among those breeds that represent this personality category are the Abyssinian, Somali, and Tonkinese.

Demonstrative

This category could also be labeled *Siamese* because that

breed represents *all* of the traits of the demonstrative personality. Cats of this type are very demanding and will follow members of their family around like an eager dog, continuing a constant flow of vocalizing. Although demonstrative cats are highly intelligent and friendly beyond belief, they complain continually if they are left alone.

Demonstrative cats are completely extroverted and do not hold back when proclaiming what they feel, what they need, or what they want. They like games and they like being the center of attention. Such cats do not like being ignored and do everything imaginable to get the attention they seem to crave so much. Cats of this category can be moody and swing from expressions of affection to actions that are highly annoying. They are capable of making the most incredible leaps from the floor to the tops of cabinets; easily open cupboard doors and refrigerators with their paws; and carry on incessant talk until they get the answers they want.

These cats are unpredictable and exhibit the most awesome behavior, from deliberately knocking something off a table to jumping into whatever you are doing at the time, all designed to get your attention. Despite all this, demonstrative cats are affectionate, fascinating, and totally devoted to their families. Representative breeds of this personality type are the Siamese and the breeds stemming from the Siamese, such as the Oriental Shorthair, Colorpoint Shorthair, Balinese, Javanese, and Tonkinese.

Timid

This is a personality trait that is not a typical characteristic of any particular breed. Many purebred and mixed-breed cats are timid.

A timid cat is usually at ease with its own family and

is comfortable at home. However, when strangers enter the house, whether they are people, dogs, or other cats, its reactions range from timidity to terror. Every time a timid cat must cope with a new person or a new situation, its insecurities and fear may come to the surface, causing it to hide under a bed or behind a couch. Some cats express their fear or anxiety by finding some place other than their litter pans to urinate or defecate.

A timid cat lacks self-confidence, views most unfamiliar situations as risky, and behaves accordingly. It may run and hide, stay in one place waiting for the intrusion to end, or very cautiously investigate a new person. Such cats are either sensitive, reserved, bashful, suspicious, distrustful, or frightened. In the extreme, a truly frightened cat may become hostile and try to defend itself, hissing, scratching, or even biting.

Timid cats are easily scared and must be treated with kindness and understanding. Their families must avoid overbearing behavior and handle the cat with gentleness and sensitivity.

Aggressive

This is another personality trait that is not a typical characteristic of any particular cat breed. There are individual purebred and mixed-breed cats that are aggressive.

The description "aggressive personality" refers to hostile-like playfulness, irritating curiosity, and pushiness, or it can refer to the behavior of a threatening cat that stalks, pounces, or even attacks another animal or a human. A cat with an aggressive personality may be endearing to its owner but terrifying to all others.

In some situations the cat's owner does not recognize this personality type for what it is and may make excuses for it. For example, some aggressive cats will hold an owner's hand or wrist between their teeth when being stroked or petted. They rarely bite down, but the danger is always present. The owner's rationale may be that this is a gesture of endearment rather than the aggressive behavior that it actually is. An aggressive cat or kitten may scratch or bite when being petted or rubbed affectionately. So-called "love bites" are indicative of an aggressive personality and should be dealt with accordingly. Cats with aggressive personalities are capable of progressing from assertiveness to intimidation and finally to menacing behavior. An aggressive cat may show hostile body language by staring at you without flinching, raising its hackles and standing directly in front of you in a crouched position that indicates it is ready to pounce or jump. Hissing and growling are warnings that an attack is imminent.

The aggressive personality can be upsetting, threatening, or dangerous. Such a cat or kitten may bite you accidentally or do it on purpose. Either way, aggressiveness must be dealt with quickly and firmly. See Chapter Seven, "Cat Problems."

3

CAT SCAN

Feline behavior, or cat psychology, is a subject that often leads to heated debates. Many feel that cats are mysterious creatures whose psyches are enigmatic, obscure, and therefore unknowable. For some, cat psychology is simply a matter of defining brain functions, the physical senses (such as vision, hearing, taste), and various reflexes. For others its roots are found in comparisons to human behavior. A widely accepted view is an area of study known as *ethology*, the biology of behavior, with an emphasis on species-typical responses in natural environments. In other words, in order to understand your cat, you must understand what your cat would be like if he were living in his natural environment, such as the mountains, deserts, or jungles. It is just possible that all the above views combined are correct.

The ethological view is that your cat's behavior, to a large extent, has been predetermined by nature and that many of his predictable responses are triggered by events in the environment as well as from learned experiences. It is based on matters pertaining to territory, hunting for food, mating, fighting to survive and so on. Despite the fact that much of this behavior is no longer necessary for survival, it is still set in motion under the right circumstances in

65

domestic cats living as pets. This tends to baffle many pet owners and often causes problems of animal/human compatibility. The contradiction between feline instincts and the lack of need for them adds to the image of the cat as a mysterious creature.

Pets can become neurotic when humans do not understand natural feline behavior and interfere with the call of the wild. Understanding your cat's natural inclinations and how to cope with them may help you avoid serious behavior problems that lead to bad endings.

Is a domestic cat normal or neurotic if he does what comes naturally when confronted with a set of circumstances that parallels a situation in the wild? For example, if a cat urinates on the floor of your home where another cat has been, is he simply being bad or is he reclaiming lost territory with his scent? Knowing why your cat does what he does helps to find a solution that is satisfactory for everyone.

Ethology, as an offshoot of zoology, has determined that normal house cats have inherited the same responses to many situations as their wild cousins exhibit. They have been genetically organized to behave in certain ways under certain conditions no matter where they are living.

Most male cats think of themselves as dominant among other cats, even though they spend most of their time alone when living in the wild. They will develop a territory, defend it if necessary, hunt for food, and fight other males for the privilege of engaging in sex. Female cats do all that, too, but do not usually fight for sexual activity. Additionally, females have the inherent drive to procreate and nurture kittens. This is all normal behavior for most cats, big or small, domestic or wild.

Loosely speaking, this is the basis on which much of so-called cat psychology rests, but too often cat behavior is confused with human psychology. Because of the complexity of the human brain and accompanying emotional system, fine lines of distinction are drawn between human behavior that is normal, eccentric, and neurotic. Certain forms of erratic human behavior are referred to as *neurosis,* which can be characterized as a disorder of the personality in which behavior is defensive and often exaggerated. The neurotic person experiences anxiety because of unconscious efforts to solve unconscious conflicts. This may cause obsessions, compulsions, hysteria, phobias, illnesses (imagined or real), loss of memory, and most serious of all, depression.

Millions of people throughout the world suffer from various forms of neuroses but manage to live with them. For some the disorder develops an implacable existence and seriously interferes with the realization of life goals, inner peace, personal happiness, and human fulfillment. Clearly, abnormal behavior is far more complicated in human beings than it is in cats. Defining abnormal *human* behavior has become as difficult as treating it therapeutically. *Cat* behavior, however, is not nearly as mysterious.

In the most general terms, it is possible that humans and cats share similar behavior mechanisms that, when disturbed, create anxiety accompanied by abnormal or neurotic responses. These fundamental disturbances may be related to attempts at obtaining or defending one's territory, creating or losing one's place in a social structure, or coping with population density. Individuals and species vary, but at some level, all creatures appear to respond in the same manner to comparable circumstances that are upsetting.

Subtlety and imagination make human neurosis enigmatic and elusive. Feline behavior is very clear, for the most part, in its normal state and equally clear in its abnormal or neurotic state. When a person has a grasp of natural feline behavior, then he or she can more readily understand when the family cat is not behaving in a normal way. With this information, solving behavior problems then becomes possible. See Chapter Seven, "Cat Problems."

The Senses

Understanding natural cat behavior promotes a healthy, happy relationship between humans and their feline pets. Therefore it is necessary to see the connection between the physical responses caused by the cat's sensory organs and its patterns of behavior. When attempting to understand the inner workings of even the most ordinary cat, it is useful to grasp the complexities of the cat's sensory organs because of their profound influence on behavior. In a very real sense, your cat's survival depends on the information provided by the senses of sight, sound, smell, taste, and touch. Sensory information is received and then conveyed to the brain by the eyes, the ears, the nose, the mouth, the skin, and the whiskers.

Sight

Sight can be explained as a sensory experience that occurs when light rays pass through the eyes (or photoreceptor organs), stimulate connective nerves, and send signals to the brain. As in a computer, these signals are electrical pulses containing information. The brain translates the pulses and interprets them into the language of thought or, in the case of animals, into pure subjective information. Vision is fixed to understanding what is seen. The difference in vision between humans and cats is how the visual information supplied to the brain is interpreted. That is an aspect of the visual experience where cats and humans part company. For example, when small objects move quickly past the cat's line of vision, they automatically elicit a set of hunting behaviors. Obviously, humans do not respond in the same way.

Of all its senses, sight provides the cat with its most extraordinary capability. Each eye can encompass a wide range of vision, and when enhanced by the mobility of the head, a cat can explore a vast horizon and always be ready to defend itself. The field of vision is measured by the portion seen by both eyes, the portion that can only be seen by one eye on each side, and the portion unseen behind the head. The cat has a large binocular field of 120 degrees directly in front of it, with a relatively small uniocular area of 80 degrees to each side. The blind area in back of the head accounts for approximately 80 degrees. Cats probably cannot focus on close objects very well, but beyond seven feet nothing escapes their view.

For many, the eyes of a cat are the most striking feature, and perhaps the most beautiful. For those who really understand these creatures, feline eyes are even more extraordinary for their special abilities than their good looks. The eyes of the cat are dramatically large and reflect how important vision is for these animals. In daylight they have about the same visual sharpness as humans. However, a cat's sensitivity to low light levels is about six times greater than a human's, which allows the cat's eyes to adjust to sudden darkness faster than ours.

Inside and to the rear of the cat's eye is the retina, which receives light and sends it to the brain as vision. Behind it is a layer of cells known as the *tapetum lucidum*. Its function is to reflect any light not absorbed during the first passage through the retina. This second pass of low light allows cats to see clearly in near darkness, which is when they usually go on the hunt for mice and other prey animals. When you see your cat's eyes glow in the dark, it is the reflection of light striking the iridescent cells of the *tapetum lucidum*.

Each eye contains a third eyelid commonly called the *haw*. It protects the eye by sliding horizontally across the surface when the eye is closed, which is why we rarely see it. When not covering the lens, it is at rest within the inner corner of the eye near the nose.

Smell

Although the nose is part of the respiratory system, it also houses the olfactory nerves which provides the sense of smell. The sense of smell is associated with securing and selecting food, avoiding predators, and facilitating various social behaviors, particularly those involving sex and reproduction. Smell is an important tool for protection as well as appetite. Cats can smell better than humans but not as well as dogs.

The sense of smell in cats is very well developed. It functions within the nasal cavity, which is enclosed by bone and cartilage and is divided in half by a vertical plate composed of bone and cartilage with a mucous membrane cover. Within the nasal cavity there are numerous rolled structures called *conchae* and *turbinates*. These structures provide a greater surface area to aid in filtering, warming, and humidifying the inhaled air before it enters the lungs. The sense of smell originates in olfactory nerves located in the turbinates, septum, and sinuses.

Each time air is inhaled, a complex series of mechanisms is set into motion. Inhaled air passes through the nose, pharynx (back of nose and upper throat), and larynx (lower portion of throat) into the trachea, which divides at its lower end into two main passages leading to the right and left lungs.

Above the upper palate of the mouth is a pouchlike organ called the *vomeronasal organ*, or organ of Jacobson, which opens into the mouth and nose. It has been suggested that it serves the sense of smell and taste with receptor cells similar to those in the olfactory organ and receives specific sexual pheromones, which are chemical odors in urine and glandular secretions. The sexual odors are carried to the vomeronasal organ with the aid of a behavior known as *flehmen*. It is a behavior pattern in which the mouth opens, the teeth become exposed from an upper lip curl, the nasal passages close, and the head jerks back. It has been observed by researchers in the reproductive season, after the male has licked the female's urine or vulva.

The nose is the respiratory system's first defense against harmful particles that are inhaled, such as dust, pollen, and microbes. It also plays a role in allowing the cat to create sound with its voice.

When viruses invade the feline body, they may cause the cat to temporarily lose its sense of smell. The cat may also lose its appetite for its usual ration. This can be offset by feeding the cat odorous delicacies such as organ meats, fish, or any food sprinkled with garlic powder. A loss of the sense of smell may also effect the cat's sexual behavior because it is unable to distinguish a male from a female.

Taste

Although the sense of taste is commonly associated with the savoring of food, its most important function pertains to various aspects of survival. Some researchers have suggested that the sense of taste provides signals for the value of food. There is also some evidence that selection behavior based on taste may be connected to the body's need for such necessities as salt, minerals, and various other nutrients. There are those who believe that taste has evolved in cats, permitting them to reject toxic substances and accept nutritious growths and commodities. However, this is not a widely accepted view.

The tongue is an important part of the mouth apparatus, providing the cat with the sense of taste. It also plays a vital role in the mechanics of eating and personal grooming. It is long, thin, and facile, with an abrasive surface consisting of a group of large *papillae* (nipple-like projections) which point backward on the upper surface. The tongue serves as a scraping-scooping instrument for eating and as a cleaning tool for the hair coat. It is one of the more unique features of the feline body.

The taste organs are commonly referred to as *taste buds*. Because they require a moist surface, they are distributed over and around the tongue. Taste buds are spherical nests of cells embedded in the upper layers of the tongue's surface. However, some researchers state that cats are unresponsive to or avoid most common taste substances. It has not been completely determined whether taste and/or smell play a major role in the cat's intake of food. Cats seem to have a preference for natural foods such as meat, fish, and fowl. Many experienced cat owners have observed that domestic cats prefer salty and sour foods more than sweet or bitter foods. Some owners tell of family cats that enjoy such foods as cantaloupe, ice cream, vegetables, and so on.

Although *the teeth* do not *directly* relate to the sense of taste, they are a part of the tactile mechanism and therefore are worthy of mention. They should be considered a factor in relation to that sensorial ability.

Each half of the jaw, lower and upper, contains small cutting teeth (*incisors*) and two sword-shaped, powerful *canines*. In addition, there are three *premolars* and one *molar* on each side of the upper jaw and two premolars and one molar on each side of the lower jaw. Cats bite with the sides of their mouths, not with the front. The front teeth, supported by the rough tongue, scrape meat from bones. The cat's thirty teeth are designed for stabbing, slicing, and biting. This unique aspect enables cats to be the most skilled predators in nature.

Tasting Catnip

Catnip is nature's chlorophyll cocktail. After a cat nibbles on this herbal substance, you can expect him to roll around on the floor, rub his face against your legs, jump straight in the air, leap about, and end in glossy-eyed calm. In some rare cases, cats have become slightly aggressive after a nip of the mint.

Its usual effect is to first stimulate the cat into unusual movements and antics. After ten or fifteen minutes kitty calms down and settles into an easygoing state of gratification. Those who give their cats catnip believe it to be a harmless source of fun and pleasure for their favorite companions. Many veterinarians agree with this view. But it is surprising to discover how few cat owners use catnip or even know much about this interesting plant.

Watching a cat respond to catnip for the first time can be puzzling or even alarming, but concern usually turns to amusement.

If a cat responds to catnip, and some do not, the effect is relatively short, ending in a nice, long nap. It is believed that all species of cats, from lions to pussycats, may experience the mood swing effect of catnip. However, not all cats within each species are affected by the plant.

Some experts feel that catnip is a natural herb and among the few vegetables that cats eat. They eat catnip and they eat grass, seemingly for their own well-being. Grass is eaten and regurgitated presumably to clear the digestive tract of hairballs and other undigested substances. Catnip is eaten and digested. It has been suggested that it too may aid the digestive process as well as serve as a tonic, or as a stimulant. It is definitely a mood enhancer that promotes a seemingly pleasant response in most cats. In past generations people drank catnip tea and called it *spring tonic*. In fact, catnip wasn't grown for cats until recent times. It was only grown for humans and was used as a medicinal herb, not a drug.

The relationship between the plant and the animal was not fostered by humans, but, in fact, is an observed relationship in nature. If you have a farm and you're growing catnip or if the catnip is growing wild, cats will find the plants and eat them and then roll around in them.

Catnip is not native to North America. It was brought here from Asia and Europe. In England it was originally called *the cat's mint* because domestic cats were attracted to the plant, which is a member of the mint family. In England eating something sparingly is "to nip at it." Hence, the herb's name, the cat's nip. It was brought to North America by early settlers and entered their herb gardens for human consumption.

In earlier times, before the pharmaceutical industry, catnip was a popular herbal medicine to aid digestion, generate perspiration (presumably for the cure of colds and flus), and to reduce body heat and high fevers. According to *Potter's New Cyclopaedia of Medicinal Herbs and Preparations* by R. W. Wren (Harper Colophon Books, 1972) it was taken as a hot tea by infusing one ounce of catnip with one pint of boiling water. Adults were given two tablespoonfuls of the tea, and children were given two or three teaspoonfuls frequently, to relieve pain and flatulence.

The entry for catnip in Palmer and Fowler's *Fieldbook of Natural History* (McGraw Hill, 1975) reads: "*Nepeta cataria*. Height to 3 ft. Stems erect, spreading, branched, grayish-green and lighter than most mints. Leaves opposite; dark above and light beneath, to 3 in. long, with rather deeply scalloped or notched margins, sometimes clustered close to ground, rather long-petioled [long-stemmed], not stiff, rather thick. Substantial root system . . .

"Oil extracted and used by trappers. Tops used medicinally as a mild tonic . . . Cats are affected by the plant. They eat the leaves and rub against the plant. Leaves are collected, dried, and packaged in cloth bags which are used by cats as playthings."

Catnip is sometimes misconstrued as a drug for cats offering some form of narcotic effect. Although some may hold this view, the majority of animal professionals do not.

"I think catnip, in moderation, is a wonderful treat for a cat," says Dr. Lewis Berman, one of New York City's most distinguished veterinarians. Dr. Berman is past president of the New York City Veterinary Medical Association, and he has served as a trustee for the Morris Animal Foundation.

"The difference, basically, between drugs and catnip," he says, "is that drugs are habit forming and catnip is not. The human body not only develops a tolerance for drugs such as cocaine, heroin, or even marijuana, with a need to have more and more, but the drugs also change certain cells in the body. In differentiating catnip, there has never been any report that catnip affects the animals' cells, chromosomes, internal organs such as the kidneys or liver or that the brain cells have been disturbed. The cat becomes normal soon after having a little fun with the catnip. I have seen my own cats with catnip toys. They roll with them, kick them, throw them in the air. If the catnip is in the dried flowered form they roll around in the stuff and take a little bit in their mouths. It's a cute and amusing thing for cats to play with. That's how I feel about it."

In *The Cornell Book of Cats* (Villard Books, 1990) the subject is referred to in a chapter on reproductive physiology written by Professor Donald Lein, D.V.M., Ph.D.: "Catnip leaves contain a chemical substance called Nepetalactone, which produces a characteristic behavior that simulates the antics of estrous queens [female cats in heat]. It is an olfactory response mediated by the *vomeronasal organ*. Catnip is not considered a feline sex pheromone [an aroma-producing secretion]. It is, instead, an hallucinogen that induces pleasurable behavior in cats, independent of sex or the presence of sex organs. Therefore, giving them catnip has no sexual side effects, and they enjoy it. The catnip response appears to be inherited as an autosomal dominant trait." (i.e. It is not sex-linked.)

Many experienced cat owners rub catnip on scratch posts to induce their pets to use them. Some breeders believe catnip works as an aphrodisiac and enhances sexual activity. Others believe it to be more like a sedative, calming cats that may be hyperactive or emotionally stressed.

Sound

The cat's ability to hear is far superior to the hearing of humans, even that of young children. The highest hearing range for humans is twenty kilocycles. Cats can hear between fifty and sixty kilocycles. They are capable of capturing sounds from the environment that humans are never aware of. They can hear the distant movement and vocal squeaks of mice and isolate them from other sounds. This may explain why they often ignore humans speaking to them. They may simply be distracted.

The feline ear not only supplies the cat with audio information but also provides the sense of balance and equilibrium. The ear is divided into three portions: the *external* ear, the *middle* ear, and the *internal* ear. The external ear consists of the outer ear (the *pinna* or *auricle*) and the ear canal. The middle ear consists of the eardrum and various small bones. The internal ear is enclosed within the skull and contains the sensory structures of hearing and balance.

The external ear conducts sound to the middle ear and serves to protect the middle and inner ear. The auricle projects from the head and serves to collect the vibrations of the air by which sound is produced. Unlike in humans, the cat's auricle can be turned in different positions without turning the head, using muscles connected to the external ear.

The middle ear is an irregular space within the temporal bone that is filled with air which comes to it through the auditory tube from the back of the nose. The components of the middle ear, the *tympanic membrane* (eardrum) and the *auditory ossicles* (small bones) convey vibrations from the external ear across the cavity to the internal ear. The muscles within the middle ear also protect the inner ear from injury from loud noises.

The internal ear relays the vibrations to the acoustic nerve. The labyrinth, named for its complexity of shape, is composed of semicircular canals which regulate the sense of balance and the *cochlea*, a curled bone that contains the organ of Corti, the actual organ of hearing. It is the composition of the inner ear that gives the cat its superior sense of hearing in addition to its unique sense of equilibrium, which enables it to jump nimbly, walk on narrow surfaces without falling, and adjust its body quickly and gracefully if it should fall.

Touch

The sense of touch plays an important role in every aspect of the cat's daily activities, especially with regard to survival mechanisms. It is involved in behavior pertaining to hunting, eating, mating, fighting, and so on. Along with the other senses, it contributes to the cat's ability to perceive its environment. The sense of touch is facilitated by the skin.

The skin is the largest sensory organ of the body. It provides the brain with information derived from the sense of touch. Its primary function, of course, is to serve as an outer covering of the body, providing a waterproof barrier against invasion by disease-causing life-forms. The skin also helps retain the body's moisture, thus preventing dehydration and dangerous temperature fluctuations in addition to providing insulation from extreme heat and cold. Although the feline skin is an efficient sensory organ, it is thinner and more vulnerable to injury than the skin of other animals.

The sensory surface conveys information to the brain concerning aspects of the external environment such as textures, temperatures, shapes, atmospheric conditions, closeness of other animals, pain, wounds, and all normal and abnormal physical sensations. The feline *integument* or skin cover begins with mucous membrane tissues at the natural openings of the digestive, respiratory, and urogenital tracts. The skin (*cutis*), with its two layers—the *dermis* and *epidermis*—covers the entire body, together with certain appendages or modifications such as hair, whiskers, paw pads, and claws.

The epidermis, the outer layer of the skin, contains pigment cells that establish color, helping to screen out harmful solar rays from the body. The function of the epidermis is to protect the body from external conditions by preventing the entrance of harmful substances or disease-causing microbes. This protection is achieved with a protein material called *keratin*. The epidermis consists of five layers of distinctive tissue, one of which is the hair.

The dermis is the underlying support structure directly beneath the epidermis that provides a second layer of protection from invasion or injury. The epidermis and the *cutaneous appendages* grow upon and within it and derive nourishment from it. The bulk of the dermis or connective tissue is made up of a material called *collagen*. The dermis also supports the hair follicles, sweat glands, and sebaceous glands.

For some, the cat's haircoat is its most attractive feature. It is, of course, a covering of hair. It is also an extension of the skin. The hair coat consists of three types of hair: *primary* or *guard hairs* within the outer coat; *awn hairs* (intermediate-sized hairs forming part of the primary coat); and *secondary hairs* (downy hair found in the undercoat). Guard hairs are thick, straight hairs that insulate the body, protect the skin, and support the sense of touch. Awn hairs are thinner and also insulate and protect the body. The thin secondary hairs help to regulate the temperature of the body by preventing excessive heat loss. All hairs are attached to *arrector pili* muscles. Prior to combat (even as play behavior) or in response to emotional stress, the *arrector pili* contract, causing the hair to stand erect.

The hair coat is seen in a wide variety of colors and patterns. Its length can be long, medium, or short, and is usually straight. The curly (Rex coat) or wirehaired coats are mutations identified with only a few breeds: Devon Rex, Cornish Rex, and American Wirehair.

Because of its fibrous and bulky nature, hair affords great protection against cuts, abrasions, thermal and radiation injury, and chemical irritation. It also serves as a filter and insulator. Hair prevents many harmful substances from making contact with the skin and can blunt injurious cuts, tears, and rips.

The whiskers are pressure-sensitive hairs or *vibrissae*. They are specialized tactile hairs called *sinus hair,* found on the muzzle, above the eyes, and on the underside of the lower foreleg. These hairs are thick, stiff, and tapered at the tip. When relaxed, they are held sideways. When the cat is concentrated on something, the whiskers are extended forward. It is thought that they aid the sense of touch, much like fingertips, and may be sensitive to air currents which would supply the cat with additional information. They are extremely sensitive and react to the slightest touch or pressure. The whiskers are also a mechanical measuring device that assists the cat in perceiving close objects that are potentially dangerous.

The forepaws and hindpaws are extremely important conveyers of physical sensations. They are the first parts of the cat's body to touch most surfaces. Each forepaw has five claws and five toe pads (two pads are placed higher on the leg). Each hindpaw has four claws and four pads plus a large metatarsal pad.

The thick, fatty toe pads are covered with a tough, dense layer of skin that cushions the shock caused by movement, like a pair of well-designed running shoes. Eccrine sweat glands open directly on the surface of the toe pads and promote cooling by the evaporation of their secretions. These secretions are produced in response to elevated body temperature, emotional stress, or excitation.

The toe pads are named according to which bones they protect, such as the *digital, metacarpal, carpal* (front only), and *metatarsal* (rear only). All cats walk on their toes. The pads distribute body weight equally, contributing to the graceful motion that is so notably feline.

The claws are literally extensions of the toes and play a role in conveying sensory information based on touch. In addition, the blade-like claws are the cat's most important weapons, next to his teeth. They are also designed for digging and for traction. The claws are pulled up behind the toes (retracted) as the cat walks and are drawn out like swords when he attacks. When the claws are relaxed, two pairs of elastic bands pull up the first element of each toe. The claws, which are attached to these elements, are then retracted inside a sheathlike fold of skin.

The Nature of Feline Behavior

In nine lifetimes you will never know as much about your cat as your cat knows about you. The truth of the matter is that there are precious few absolutes regarding the behavior of the domestic cat. Research, serious observation, and experience have supplied us with what little we actually know. There are no hard and fast scientific truths with regard to feline behavior that can be applied to all cats. More is known about wolf behavior and its application to the domestic dog than is known about feline behavior and its application to the domestic cat. In a sense, domestic cats make their own rules and define themselves as they go along. Novice cat owners quickly learn what the more experienced owners already know—that it is easier and more productive to understand one's self in relation to cats than to pursue absolutes of feline behavior.

Humans who live with cats have taken on the role of caretaker and it is essential for them to understand what information is available about the nature of the feline spirit. The information provided here is not offered so that the cat owner can change the family pet's nature, but rather as a guided tour through the mind of an intricate and fascinating animal. Your cat is a unique creature. He offers no apology for his uncompromising and sometimes contradictory behavior. Your choice is to try to manipulate the external conditions for a desired effect or to accept the behavior as a matter of reality.

Much of the domestic cat's basic behavior is similar if not identical to the basic behavior of most species of wild cats. The primary difference, of course, is the domestic cat's total acceptance of the conditions in the human environment. With few exceptions cats raised in the wild will not tolerate close proximity to humans, while almost all domestic cats relish the relationships they develop with humans.

It is part of the feline nature to live in self-imposed solitude, marking territory, hunting, and socializing only during mating and cub rearing. Why, then, will our pet cats tolerate life in a household with a troop of humans, dogs, and other cats?

Cats living in the wild prefer to live in solitude and do not hesitate to fight other cats when necessary. They do not make social contact except for the purpose of mating and rearing their young. And yet such solitary creatures have the capacity for developing close relationships with humans. One can only infer that the closeness with humans resembles the bond that existed between a kitten and his mother and siblings. This bond, of course, weakens and eventually severs as the kitten matures. For reasons unknown, this sense of attachment with other creatures can be continued beyond the time it normally lasts and, indeed, can even be restored in adulthood under the right circumstances. In the wild the social contacts of adult cats are fully occupied with matters pertaining to territory, defense, competition, sex, and reproduction. In other words, relationships with other cats are usually of an adversarial nature allowing no opportunity for the friendly behaviors of kittenhood.

Accordingly, long, enduring relationships between humans and domestic cats develop along lines similar to those between parent and child, or among siblings. The instant a human assumes the responsibility of feeding and caring for a cat, he or she is eliciting a form of juvenile dependency from the animal. This juvenile behavior may have always been present but in a dormant state, waiting for the proper conditions.

Without even knowing it, a kindly human family may trigger in their new kitten or adult cat the behavioral responses associated with juvenile activities. This may be because it is not necessary for the average house cat to defend himself in a typical pet home as he must in almost all other situations. Under these circumstances it is possible for cats to bond with humans and enter into lasting friendships that would never develop with other cats in a natural setting.

Taking the hypothesis one step further, we can see in the domestic cat a paradox of behavior. The skills of the solitary hunter coupled with the capabilities of an aggressive competitor produce an adult cat with instant self-sufficiency. However, the acceptance of loving care produces an eternal kitten or juvenile cat. Therefore, our beloved house cats are both independent and dependent at the same time. This may be the only difference between wild and domestic cats other than size. It may also be a bit of their mystery.

A general understanding of basic cat behavior can make life much more pleasant for those who have taken in cats as members of the family. Although some traits can be altered through environmental manipulation, the primary objective here is to understand what is *natural* or *unnatural* in the family cat's behavior. When they are understood, many characteristics of the cat cease to be objectionable and help the owner appreciate the inner qualities as well as the external aesthetics of the cat. The need to scratch, to dig around the litter box, to present a dead mouse at your feet are but a few examples.

There are several major areas of feline behavior that are most important for the cat owner to understand. Naturally these topics must, by necessity, be dealt with in abbreviated form, with the details of some aspects left out entirely. However, this introduction to cat behavior will at least open the door and give the cat lover a concise but useful understanding of what is going on with their furry friend and family member. The most important aspects of cat behavior, domestic and wild, are territory, hunting, sex and reproduction, and social behavior.

Territory

The term territory simply refers to an area an animal regularly inhabits. The animal behaves as though the area is an extension of himself; he may accept some interlopers or he may attempt to drive them away. Territory is sometimes inherited, won in combat, or discovered and claimed after its abandonment by a previous animal.

Territory is not always a fixed bit of real estate. Sometimes it is simply the area that an animal claims during a given season or a particular time of the day. For cats, however, territories are loosely fixed areas influenced by time, space, and other creatures.

We are told by Edward O. Wilson in *Sociobiology:* "Nearly all vertebrates and a large number of the behaviorally most advanced invertebrates, conduct their lives according to precise rules of land tenure, spacing, and dominance. These rules mediate the struggle for competitive superiority. They are enabling devices that raise personal or inclusive genetic fitness." In other words, territory is claimed and defended (often aggressively) out of an inherent drive for the purpose of species or individual survival. Most mammals instinctively struggle for territory in order to protect their food supply. These instincts for territory are especially imbued in the cat. Despite the many generations of domesticity in the typical house cat, the instinct to claim and defend territory is quite strong.

There are two important locations that define a cat's territory. The first is the *core area* or *immediate home,* which receives the heaviest use. The immediate home area is where most daily activities take place. It also contains the lair, the safest sleeping area in the entire territory. In domesticity, the core area may be an entire house, one room in an apartment, or perhaps a portion of a room. The second location is the *home* or *outer range.* This is a vague, loosely defined area composed of interconnecting pathways and trails leading to water, resting places, scent posts (marked by the cat with urine or scratches), emergency retreats, and favorite sunning spots. It is also where most hunting takes place. The home range may be an entire valley or portion of a mountain range for some of the larger cats. For domestic cats it may be a basement, a kitchen, a back alley, or a yard.

Male cats claim larger territories than females. Female cats are especially intolerant of territorial intrusions from other female cats. Quite frequently the outer ranges of neighboring cats overlap, a situation that is tolerated because the territoriality of cats also has to do with time. Neighboring cats may hunt the same terrain but at different times. They will try to avoid each other at all costs. This scheduling of use of space prevents confrontations and fighting. It is quite a different situation from the sharing of common territory by two or more cats who live with a human family. Here an informal order of rank and superiority coupled with the cats' juvenile tendencies help maintain order and a pleasant atmosphere.

Animal behavior regarding territory varies from casual to intense. All cats, wild and domestic, have strong sets of responses concerning the acquisition and defense of territory. Domestic cats rarely have the opportunity to choose their territory. Even so, once they are brought to a place, they relate to it as their wild cousins do. Animals who graze in a herd (e.g., wildebeests) and those who hunt in a pack (e.g., wolves) travel vast distances in a sprawling, ill-defined territory, creating a great overlap of ranges. Consequently their attitude toward territory is much more casual than that of cats.

With the exception of lions, cats in the wild live and hunt alone. Their hunting techniques involve stalking and ambushing, lunging and pouncing. Their territories are smaller and more exclusive than those of other mammals. Few cats in the wild can afford to tolerate an incursion into their territory by another cat. This fact is of vital importance to cat owners because it explains why their pets may become upset with a new cat, a human they do not trust, visiting cats, or a move to a new house. From the family cat's point of view, any change affecting territory is a threat to its sense of survival.

These tendencies are made apparent by the degree of emotion shown when the cat's territory is violated or moved. The most common expression of emotional distress is to urinate and defecate in various parts of the new premises (read: territory) instead of in the litter box. Sometimes the cat behaves as though it is depressed (and it may well be). An unhappy cat may make low, throaty sounds you never heard before and might even start clawing the furniture, the walls, the curtains, or the nearest person. Although relationships with humans and other animals become very important to domestic cats, loss of territory is of greater importance. It is taken as a catastrophe. While a domestic cat assumes it will survive without you, instinct indicates that the cat is in jeopardy with the loss of established territory. This grievous fear is usually not based in fact, because the human has simply exchanged one territory for another. But the cat doesn't know this; it takes great patience and much extra attention to convince the cat he is still safe when he is uprooted from his territory and moved somewhere else.

An extremely important aspect of territory for the cat owner to understand has to do with *marking*. This refers to the acts by which a cat in the wild or at home leaves his mark or individual sign of identity in various parts of the immediate home or the home range, or on another cat's territory. Researchers are not sure of the reasons for territory marking and can only offer educated guesses.

Some believe it is used as a boundary demarcation so that wandering or visiting cats will know they are trespassing. However, few cats have ever been reported to turn in the opposite direction on coming upon a territory mark. It may be a guide for cats to avoid each other, and thus prevent sudden clashes. Another aspect of territory marking is message sending with a special function for mating, a perfumed love letter, so to speak.

Territory marking is accomplished in several ways. The most common and least understood by new cat owners has to do with the cat's toileting habits. All cats, male and female, *spray* as a means of marking. When a cat marks territory or asserts itself, closely related motives, he may spray urine against some vertical object, defecate, scratch or claw something, paw wipe, or vocalize. Quite often more than one of these methods are employed at the same time. This information can be of some help to the cat owner who doesn't understand why the family cat has suddenly "gone berserk" with unacceptable behavior.

It has been thought for a long time that the spraying of urine by male cats is eliminated once the animal has been castrated. This is one of the primary reasons pet owners are advised to have this surgical procedure done. Information from experienced cat owners indicates this is not necessarily the case. Altering a male usually but not always prevents spraying. One must consult a veterinarian for more complete information.

Most male cats (and some females) at various times will back up against a wall, a window, a piece of furniture, or some outdoor object and spray urine against it. In the case of unaltered male cats this urine usually is quite pungent and upsets everyone who comes in contact with it. Sometimes cats rub their faces in it and then rub against other objects. Every breed of cat, every species of cat, behaves in this manner. It is the most common form of marking, although defecation is also used for this purpose. Spraying may also be a form of sexual communication by either male or female.

Spraying urine and/or defecating can also be used by a cat as a sign of defiance to another cat after a nonviolent confrontation. This will occur at various spots already sprayed in the past as territory marks. In a litter box, the feces is usually buried beneath the sand. But on occasion the cat will bury the old feces and display the new feces on top of a mound of sand. This may be accompanied with a throaty sound and a mad dash from room to room. Sometimes the form of running is in a stiff, sideways gait that is not unlike the cat's arched display when preparing for a showdown with another cat.

Marking territory or communicating the cat's presence is all too often accomplished by clawing visible scratches into a vertical object such as a tree, if you're lucky, or the arm of a sofa, if you're not. Although most scratching has to do with the need to remove the outer sheath of the claws, much of it has to do with assertion and the marking of territory.

Probably the most fascinating form of marking is vocal assertion. The large cats of the jungles and plains are the greatest of the vocalizers, but do not underestimate the domestic cat's powerful ability to manifest his roar. Vocalizing occurs between rival males when competing for a female in heat. There is much vocalization when two males are about to fight for territory. Sometimes vocalizing seems a lonely, haunting sound aimed at the sky, but is in fact aimed at the near and far competition.

Hunting

It is not yet known if cats stalk, kill, and eat prey animals simply because they are hungry or as an automatic reaction to seeing the animals. Researchers are not even certain if such a seemingly automatic reaction is learned or at least affected by experience. What is known is that all cats are intensely curious about scratching and high-pitched squealing noises. These stimuli do not necessarily have to be associated with any specific prey animal. Acoustic stimuli do not necessarily elicit prey catching but simply the desire for prey catching. The cat quickly moves to the source of the sound and investigates visually. All the hunting mechanisms, such as stalking, shift into gear at the first sighting of movement or sooner, if the cat is an experienced hunter.

A young, inexperienced cat tends to regard all creatures as fellow cats. A cat and a mouse placed together do not necessarily automatically play out hunter/hunted roles. If the mouse moves slowly, it will be sniffed but tolerated. However, if the mouse runs away from the cat swiftly, in a straight line, the cat will chase it and pounce upon it. This is true of any smaller animal running away from or at right angles to the cat. Conversely, when a smaller animal runs *to* the cat, the cat will hesitate and perhaps retreat. The cat's catching action is innately released by specific forms and directions of movement. Only prey with fur or a furlike covering will elicit a killing bite. The prey's scent seems to have little or no bearing on stalking or killing. Scent is used by the cat primarily for the purposes of mating and ingesting food, although experienced cats are drawn to the dried urine spots left behind by mice as they run, and cats will sniff along this type of trail.

Cats have a remarkable memory for the places they have been. A cat that experiences a hunting triumph at a particular location will remember that exact place and return again and again seeking another triumph, even after a long time lapse. This is an extremely important part of the cat's superb hunting ability and has obvious survival value.

Domestic cats can interact with captured prey in a manner that is sometimes construed as "cruel" or "heartless." It is behavior that is difficult to reconcile with the image of the pet cat who is cuddly and lovable. Cats appear to "play" with their captured prey until it mercifully dies. This instinctive behavior is programmed genetically and meant to be performed in front of kittens. Its purpose is to elicit the correct responses in kittens so that their hunting instincts will develop properly. Nature does not take into account the pet food industry or whether a male or female cat actually has kittens to teach. Both novice and experienced cat owners must understand that cats are *natural* creatures who behave with a strong survival instinct. Most living organisms have built into their behavior the drive to ensure the survival of their species. This is why most animals protect and teach their young what they know. Try to bear this in mind if you happen to witness your cat's behavior with captured prey. Consider what the captured animal probably does with *its* prey.

What constitutes the prey of domestic cats can be reduced to one simple rule: *A cat will be attracted to any living animal no bigger than itself.* Depending on the cat's aggressive inclinations, it is mostly interested in mice and rats. (It is important to note that few domestic cats will attack a full-grown Norway rat, which is the most common rat in the world.) Domestic cats are interested in most insects, including houseflies, beetles, crickets, and grasshoppers. They are also interested in frogs, toads, lizards, snakes, rabbits, shrews, moles, squirrels, and birds. With regard to birds a reassuring note to bird and cat lovers is the fact that cats are capable of catching only old, sick, or very young avian creatures. Only on rare occasions do cats capture mature, healthy birds. What is often not appreciated is that at least three-fourths of all birds die as a result of nature's own control of the population/territory ratio. The primary factors that keep a bird population of any area relatively constant are cold weather, insufficient food, and disease. Cats could not survive if they relied on a diet of birds exclusively.

In fact, cats perform a selective function when they prey on unprotected, old, sick, or injured birds. By selecting out these birds from the population, they enhance the survival of the general population of birds. And, as stated above, the most common prey of the domestic cat is the mouse.

His method of catching his prey is what makes the cat, both domestic and wild, the consummate hunter of the entire animal kingdom. A cat usually hears his prey as the first signal. In a crouched posture he runs toward the sound. He then stops and observes in a special close-to-the-ground position. In the natural setting he would crouch behind grass, earth mounds, or other forms of cover. His principal technique is to ambush the prey animal before it has the opportunity to escape. In a stooped-shoulder manner the cat waits for the prey to move or show itself. Domestic cats are quite patient and are capable of waiting long periods. Once the prey is sighted, the cat employs a stalking run, which again is very low to the ground. This enables it to get closer to the prey without having to give chase. More observation takes place as the claws unsheathe; the tail lies flat and twitches from side to side at the tip, and the leg muscles contract in readiness to spring. Every sense the cat possesses goes into full operation, from extended whiskers to forward-pointing ears. With a wobbling motion of the hind legs, the cat prepares to attack. He springs forward, low to the ground, and bounds to the victim in a shallow leap. The cat almost always catches the mouse with its paws at this stage.

If the pounce is unsuccessful, a chase ensues, with all the advantage going to the cat. Once the mouse is caught, the cat strikes it from behind, on the back and shoulder, with one paw and holds it while the cat delivers a killing bite in front of the holding paw, directly on the nape of the prey's neck. This usually severs the spinal cord, effecting instant death. In the natural setting (and sometimes the domestic one as well), the cat then commences to eat the animal.

Experienced cat owners know that not every cat will chase, catch, kill, and eat mice. A domestic cat may perform none or one or any combination of these predatory elements. Although there is no way to be sure why this is true, there are some possible explanations for this behavior (or lack of it). It is important to recognize that every cat has the inherent tendency to hunt for food. Whether or not these instincts are developed fully depends on several factors. This behavior must be elicited at an early age by the mother, by the litter mates, and by prey itself. However, even if there is no early elicitation of the prey-catching behavior, it will appear later with the onset of hunger or with the appearance of prey animals acting in a manner that provokes this behavior.

The first prey-catching movement is made by a kitten at about three weeks of age. This is a tentative forward grope with one paw, which is also how an adult cat investigates any new, fairly small object. Lying in wait, chasing, stalking, the stalking run, and the pounce onto the prey appear in rapid succession. These are completely developed by the time the mother cat brings the first live prey animals, usually mice, to the kittens, in about their sixth week. This is actually part of the weaning process. In the fourth week the mother cat begins to carry dead prey into the nest, where the kittens watch her eat it. In the following weeks the kittens' reactions to the prey animal mature. Thus when the mother brings the first live mouse into the nest, the kittens have at their disposal all of the instinctive movements for prey catching. The killing bite is the last element to develop. This late development has survival value, for the kittens would surely injure one another while playing at prey catching if the response developed earlier. As they play with the first live prey animals brought into the nest by the mother, the ordered sequence leading to the killing—lying in wait, stalking, pouncing, and—establishes itself gradually, though occasionally it can happen quite suddenly.

Mother cats with kittens older than three weeks usually catch considerably more prey than at other times. This, we may presume, is for the benefit of the kittens, who are now being weaned from breast milk to partially solid food. It is the behavior of the kittens themselves that stimulates the mother's hunting activity. From the fourth to the sixth weeks the mother brings dead prey animals to the nest and growls to attract the attention of the kittens. The growling may change into a coaxing purr and she will paw the dead animal several times before eating it, once she is certain that the kittens are watching. This very same behavior can be seen in domestic cats who do not have kittens. They may catch a mouse, kill it, and then bring it to the feet of the human companion, who in this instance serves as a substitute kitten. Males as well as females behave in this manner. It is less important for the human to "congratulate" the cat than it is simply to approach the cat and look at what it caught.

Interestingly, the killing bite is not taught by the mother, but rather elicited by the mother's behavior or that of a litter mate. A live prey animal is brought into the nest and released by the mother. She swiftly catches the released mouse as the kittens observe her. They do not learn from her example, as one would imagine; their inherent instincts to give chase and to capture the prey are triggered by the mother's behavior. She appeals to their sense of competition as they eventually try to beat her to the released prey during the several times it is released. The released prey elicits the kittens' prey-catching activity by running away, and its swift recapture by the older cat compels the kittens to be even quicker if they want to catch the prey before the mother seizes it again. This is what provides the needed excitation that leads to the killing bite. It is important to note that the keenest domestic cats never seize their prey with as much wild eagerness and determination as young male wild cats. (This is what makes them suitable as pets.) Yet the instinct to kill prey is often observed by the ninth week in domestic kittens.

If the mother cat does not bring live prey to the kittens during the critical period between their sixth and about their twentieth weeks the kittens either do not kill prey later in life or else learn to do so slowly and laboriously.

The development of the killing bite is connected with the growth of the canine teeth, which are the ones employed for this purpose. The deciduous or milk teeth are all in place by the fifth week and ready to function. During the transition from deciduous to permanent teeth, there may be one or two weeks when the temporary canines are too weak to function and the permanent ones are not yet long enough. This happens sometime between the fourth and sixth months. In a natural setting the litter of kittens breaks up as a family by the sixth month. This happily coincides with the development of all the permanent teeth.

One further statement on prey capture is essential for the owner of a domestic cat: *All cats, both young and old, engage in play activity.* Much of this play behavior is connected in one way or another with prey-catching activity. For reasons partially explained above, cats tend to play with their captured prey, both before and after they have killed it. In the true play that cats indulge in (*without* prey animals), one can observe the various aspects of prey capture with or without toys or other animals. Here we often see a form of overflow energy involving all aspects of hunting and prey capture. Some cat owners refer to these energized spurts as the "nightly crazies," when the normally quiet animal suddenly dashes across the room in a crouched position. All elements of prey capture can be seen, including stalking, watching posture, creeping, pouncing, seizing with the teeth, carrying around, and tossing objects away. During the "crazies," more energy may be expended than if the cat or kitten were actually hunting real prey animals. To the novice cat owner this is a startling and perplexing set of behaviors. It is probably safe to assume that all cat play mimics the dynamics of cat existence, from prey capture to declarations of dominance to fighting over females and territory. It is harmless, fascinating, and more often than not, quite funny if not outright lovable.

Sex

To the uninitiated, feline sexuality comes as a rude and frightening shock. It creates the impression of pain, emotional trauma, and uncontrollable body disfunction for the cat. The poor loving humans stand by and agonize over their cat's great illness. Although some cats do get hurt in the process, particularly those males that must compete, there is a natural order at work that all felines must conform to—indeed, they cannot avoid it. However, it is of the utmost importance for cat lovers to understand that neither male nor female cats are sick or in pain when they lock into the cyclical compulsions connected with the mating procedure. It only looks that way.

When considering cat behavior, it is impossible to ignore sexual urges and the drive to mate. Although the biological imperative of most living organisms is to procreate, it is the furthest thing from the mind of sexually aroused cats. It would seem that the principal drive in all unaltered cats is to experience sex as frequently as possible. Females in heat and males aware of such females can think of nothing but the consummation of their potent urges. Because so much of the feline personality is overshadowed at these times by sexual appetite, it is of vital concern to the cat owner to become aware of the details of this behavior. This may help in deciding to have the male or female cat surgically sterilized, which is the best option for cat owners.

Whole male cats (tomcats) exhibit great frustration if they are not permitted to mate as often as their bodies dictate. Sexually frustrated males become hostile, restless, sometimes dangerous. They yowl and pace and spray their areas with an altogether unpleasant-smelling urine. A frustrated tomcat makes the worst possible pet or home companion. Purebred male cats that are part of an intelligent breeding program *should* be mated on a regulated basis, providing it is controlled by a responsible, informed breeder.

Unspayed females (queens) who are sexually aroused and not permitted to satisfy themselves are equally unpleasant to be around. Their vocalizing is continual, as are their physical entreaties to be allowed outdoors. In some instances unmated females remain in a constant state of heat. This can mean a nonstop display of vocalizations, rubbing, purring, and rolling behavior, in addition to odorous glandular secretions deposited anywhere from the litter box to the carpet.

Sex between cats is less violent when arranged by experienced, knowledgeable breeders. Here, a desired genetic selection is being sought in order to further the best qualities of two lines of a pure breed. The union is less violent because the female is presented to only one male and the encounter is on the male's own territory. The female cat is always brought to the male. Random matings of feral cats or cats that are permitted to roam outdoors are always violent, noisy, and somewhat bizarre to the human sensibility.

When the female goes into heat, most of the male cats in the area smell and hear her condition and become attracted and aroused. A collection of males begins to assemble around the lusty female. They travel through other cats' territories to get to the female, which sometimes causes violent confrontations. Although there may be a loosely formed order of dominance among the cats of the immediate vicinity, it is not honored by those of other areas. This creates a situation much like a time bomb. It will definitely explode. The question is when.

The female will ward off any male advances until she is quite ready for copulation. Until then the competition for her attention will intensify. One or more males will begin to circle, and then the fights begin. One, two, three, or even more tomcats may engage in savage fighting with unsheathed claws and slashing teeth, causing the most awful injuries to one another.

The males confront one another with spiky coats and arched backs, and hiss, spit, and growl. After a choreography of slow approaches accompanied by threatening vocalizations ranging from growls to shrieks, one tomcat will finally spring at another and aim his teeth at the nape of the neck as though he were after a prey animal. They slash and claw at each other, rolling furiously about, screaming and spitting. Suddenly they will break apart and move away for a needed rest. After a brief pause they will return for another confrontation, and repeat this blistering ritual several times until finally one of the participants does not return to the fight, thus accepting defeat. The fascinating element is that the victor does not always win the female. As the most dominant males are fighting, there may be one lower-ranking male who begins the courtship and quickly enjoys the female's favors while the others are still sorting themselves out in the fray.

The courtship between the male and the female cat is highly ritualized. There is the traditional pursuit and avoidance. He follows her, but she moves away. If he fails to follow, she stops and entices him with alluring gestures, rubbing, rolling, and soft purring. If the male approaches too quickly or not at the correct moment, the female rebuffs him with hissing and spitting and a swipe with her paw. A nervous or impatient female is capable of rendering painful damage to a pursuing tomcat.

Once the female is ready, she will crouch, rub her body against the ground, and cozy up to the male. She may even tread or knead with her feet as she lowers the front of her body and raises the rear in a presenting posture. Her tail is shifted to one side, giving the male complete access to the entrance to her vagina (vulva). At this point the male pounces as if she were prey, seizes her by the nape with a slight holding bite, and mounts her. He grasps her abdomen with his two front paws as his penis emerges from its protective sheath (prepuce). His hind legs hold her in place as he attempts to make entry. Both male and female keep shifting positions to facilitate this. Several attempts are made until it is accomplished. Upon entry, ejaculation *and ovulation* take place within five to fifteen seconds. The male instantly pulls away, causing the barbs on the tip of his penis to tear some inner tissue slightly. It is believed that this sensation, be it intense pain or pleasure, creates a violent reaction in the female. She emits a screaming sound, frees herself from the male grip, and attempts to strike him with a slashing claw. Most often the experienced male springs away just in time to avoid injury. Both male and female will then relax and start over again within a short time.

They may copulate as many as five or ten times in thirty minutes. The mating process can continue for twenty-four hours or even longer. During this time the male may tire of the female and allow the other waiting males to continue satisfying her needs. The female is almost certain to become pregnant, because copulation stimulates ovulation (release of an egg from the ovary) in the female. Because ovulation occurs with each mating, and because more than one male may mate with a female in heat, it is possible for the kittens of a single litter to have different genetic fathers. Wondrous are the ways of feline reproduction.

Whole male cats will mate at almost any time, especially if they are on their own territory. A free-roaming tom will travel relatively great distances to "visit" a female in heat. Mature male cats must gratify their sexual appetites or suffer severe frustration.

Mature females (between three and nine months of age, depending on the breed) experience estrus several times a year, usually between late winter and early spring. Some cats go into season more or less frequently, depending on the breed or the cat's living conditions. Climate and the ratio of daylight to darkness (including artificial light in the home) influence the frequency of estrus cycles. A cat living in artificial light in a human environment may create the conditions for sexual activity at any time of the year.

To those unprepared for it, feline sexuality is a disturbing surprise, to say the least. The human family agonizes over what they think is traumatic and painful for the cat. Often novice cat owners do not even know what they are looking at and contact the veterinarian, thinking they have a medical emergency.

The most logical response for humans to this behavior is the surgical sterilization of their pets. The term used is *neutering*. Male cats are *castrated* or *altered*, while female cats are *spayed* or given *ovariohysterectomies*. Depending on when the cat is neutered, many or most of the sexual behavior will never develop. It is best to have males altered at or before six months of age. Females should be spayed at the age of six months or older. At this writing active research and serious experimentation is being conducted on the effectiveness and safety of surgically neutering young kittens.

Most kittens are born because of free-roaming cats that are not restrained by the limitations of confinement or sexual altering. Far too few cat owners understand the sexuality of their pets. They inadvertently permit unwanted pregnancies or create tremendous sexual frustration by locking their animals away during periods of sexual urgency.

There can be no doubt that domestic cats are better off when they are sexually altered. Males and females should not be permitted to mate for any reason, especially not for profit or sex education. Cats that are mated by registered breeders and exhibitors are purebred specimens that have been genetically selected over a period of years for their special qualities of physical and mental perfection. These are developed by members of the Cat Fancy who own and operate catteries in a humane and professional manner.

An altered cat will never experience sexual frustration or the rigors of backyard mating. Life is certainly much more pleasant for the humans involved as well. A castrated male cat will not have a need or desire to wander far from home or become involved in many horrible fights resulting in cuts, bruises, or inevitable swelled abscesses on the body. The castrated male is also less likely to spray the walls of his home with the acrid odor of sexually scented urine (unless he feels the need to assert his territorial rights). Primarily, he will not impregnate a female and thus add to the already overloaded pet population.

The spayed female will cease to experience the cycles of estrus throughout the year once she has had her operation. There will be no attractant odors, no radical behavior changes, and no disturbing groans. All activities associated with reproduction will cease. However, the personality of the animal does not change, nor does any other aspect of behavior. And she will always appear to be someone special to her owners, even if she is no longer a sex goddess.

Social Behavior

A chance encounter. When two strange cats meet, which almost never happens in the wild (except for mating), they cautiously sniff each other. They investigate the immediate area, using sight, sound, and smell. They then turn back to each other. At first they appear to sniff each other's noses, although they do not actually touch. The whiskers act as feelers as they size up each other's nape and flanks and ultimately smell each other's anus. Although there is a slight resistance to this aspect of the investigation, one finally allows the other to continue smelling, provided the encounter remains friendly. Very often the friendliness ends when one moves a bit too quickly while examining the nape of the neck. Defensive postures quickly develop, and one or both begin to hiss. From there the more assertive of the two will deliver a blow on the nose with his paw and send his opponent running. This automatically establishes a kind of social structure, with one cat dominant over the other. The encounter may repeat itself several times before the confrontation ends. Depending on the territoriality of the dominant cat, things may go very sour and result in a direct physical attack. This is highly likely if both cats are whole tomcats. The cat who is on his own territory is usually the dominant animal, at least in the beginning. In variations of this behavior, both animals will crouch, staring at each other for long periods. Extremely timid cats will run and hide as long as there is a strange cat in their territory.

Fighting. Adult male cats are the most likely to fight one another. However, all cats, including those that have been neutered, are capable of engaging in combat with one another. Young cats are the least likely to engage in serious fights, although kittenish play is a foreshadowing of future aggressive behavior. When kittens fight, it is amusing to watch because of their inept techniques and because it seems more like play than combat.

Cat fights must be taken seriously and avoided at all costs because of the dangers involved to the adversaries. When cats fight, they do not have in their repertoire of behavior a gesture of submission, as do dogs, wolves, and many other mammals. This leaves a losing cat with no reasonable means of surrender and release from the fight. His only chance is to escape if possible. Frequently the winning cat chases the loser and brings him down once again. Serious injury is a certainty and may, in some situations, continue to the death. Veterinarians are often called upon to treat seriously wounded cats, with part of an ear or tail bitten off or a large abscess festering on the back of the neck.

Cats who live together. The factors that permit cats to get along with one another are not fully understood. Many experienced cat owners have perfectly delightful stories of cats who spend entire lifetimes together in peace and harmony. However, the dominance of one cat over another is usually subtle in manner and sometimes imperceptible to the enthusiastic cat lover, who translates animal actions into human terms. The use of the food bowls and litter box by a dominant cat can act as a guide to the degree of harmony in a multi-cat home. In some hierarchical structures, a top cat emerges, along with one or more low cats on the totem pole who behave in a cowering manner to all the others. One can never predict with certainty how the social structure will be developed between cats. It depends on the individual character of each of the animals involved. In some households the cats never develop a community with one dominant cat and one that is the lowest in rank. In some feline communities there are dominant cats, cats of lower rank, and even one or more social outcasts.

When two or more cats share a territory or a common home, only the gentlest form of dominance and subordination may manifest itself. Here are cats completely accustomed to one another without much need for the type of violent fights that cats are capable of engaging in. However, a strange cat entering that established society will certainly be examined and quite likely attacked. At the very least, one or more cats may express their dismay by urinating and defecating in inappropriate areas, outside their litter boxes.

Because domestic cats do not select their primary territory, but rather have it selected for them by humans, they seem to accept one another with much greater ease than their wild cousins. This is an extremely important aspect of domesticity. The denial of the primary decision in a cat's life probably has a subordinating effect. This may be what allows them to share a territory in domesticity with one or more cats.

Cat owners can greatly enhance their own and their cats' lifestyles by understanding and accepting the basics of cat behavior. The importance of territory applies to such everyday elements as feeding dishes, litter boxes, resting areas, toys, and hiding places. Allowing for predatory behavior, if only in the manner of play, is extremely important for the mental health of a house cat. Do not discourage prey capture in any form unless it is destructive to the home or someone living in it. Sexual behavior cannot be avoided unless the animal is surgically sterilized, and even then not all of it can be eliminated. Matters of dominance, social harmony, and aggressiveness must be dealt with sympathetically. By studying a cat's behavior, one cannot help but comprehend his true nature and love him all the more. It is here that you will begin to perceive the dignity of your cat.

4

A CAT IN THE FAMILY

People are highly social creatures and do their best when they live in a family style. Of course, our definition of *family* has changed drastically. We no longer think exclusively of mother, father, and children when we try to characterize a family. A family can be a mother and a daughter. A nephew and an aunt. Two friends, two lovers, or one person and a cat. We now accept the idea that a family is simply two or more creatures sharing their lives. A cat's need for family life does not seem to be as great as a dog's, judging from his solitary existence when living in the wild.

Nevertheless, cats do need their human families because of the state of dependency we have created in them over the many generations of domesticity. Cats that live as pets have been brought up to be eternal kittens and adolescents, depending on us to feed them and keep them out of trouble in the human environment. Every instinctive behavior that cats are born with is designed to help them survive on their own, after they have left their mothers and litter mates and gone off to live in a wild state. *But* . . . bringing a cat into your home prolongs the state of kittenhood indefinitely. It continues the cat's life in an artificial nest along with artificial litter mates and even an artificial mother. That's you, or more accurately, the human family.

The point is, your best opportunity for living a relatively problem-free existence with your cat is to provide him with a protected family life. And that involves understanding how your pet fits in as a member of the family. Whatever the conditions are in your family, they will have an effect on the quality of your pet's life. For better or for worse, the cat you have taken in, like the child you have borne, the spouse you have committed to, or the friend you live with, is a part of your life now. No matter what your reason was for getting a cat, its impact on every member of the family is great. The friendship, love, and responsibility of a pet cat is a shared experience for everyone involved.

Creating a Good Cat in the Family

In a family people bond together, form social attachments, develop an order of rank and privilege, work for common goals, and are concerned with survival both as individuals and as a group. It is not terribly different for animals living in the wild. We all know that cats, at various times in their lives, do the same. This may be why we are so attracted to them. We have a great deal in common with them. But unlike cats, humans join *special* families such as clubs, organizations, social groups, and cliques of friends. At times we go it alone, only to return again to one or all of our *special* families.

We band together out of our common interests, our need for other people, for companionship, for intimacy, and out of our need for a bit of comfort, warmth, and security. As John Lennon wrote, "I get by with a little help from my friends." Make no mistake about it, we all need our families, no matter what kind they are, and so do cats.

You could say that a family is simply two or more living creatures sharing their lives. For better or for worse that's what a family is about, and a cat will always fit into the equation. Our concern here is how to successfully make a cat part of your family.

Ask yourself, why do you need a cat, anyway? Protection? Hardly. Companionship? Possibly. But for many the true reason is to have one more presence in their lives to love. This is probably why we have babies. When we get a new cat, we act like proud new parents and show off the newest member of the family as if it is a blessed event. Is getting a new cat anything at all like having a baby? In some respects it is and in others there is no similarity at all.

Babies and kittens are both helpless and totally dependent on us. Babies and kittens need to be protected from themselves. That is why we *baby*-proof a house and we *kitten*-proof a house, getting rid of dangling electric cords and all the rest of it. Babies and kittens are adorable, huggable, lovable, enchanting, enticing, playful, demanding, noisy, irritating, and both manage to keep us awake at all hours of the night.

Are there any differences between them? You better believe there are. A kitten will never, never grow up, go off to college, and show up unexpectedly with six friends for dinner and twelve loads of dirty laundry. A kitten won't do that to you. Of course a kitten also won't throw its graduation cap in the air, look its parents in their teary eyes, and say, "Thanks, Mom and Dad, for this diploma." However, a kitten *will* grow into a cat and love you, adore you, and stay with you till the end.

The principal difference between children and kittens is their view of the world. Children struggle to understand the world so they can reshape it for their own purposes. This is a normal part of the process of growing up. Kittens grow into cats accepting the world without question and trying to live in harmony with it. That is an enormous difference. Therein lies the clue for making your cat a good cat in the family. It all has something to do with harmony and it's so easy.

So how do you get a new cat to enter family life with ease, comfort, and success? There are three elements involved. They are

1. Understanding natural cat behavior
2. Bonding with your cat
3. Getting your cat under your control

That's it. That's all there is to it. It's simple enough, but God help you and your cat if you don't do that much. You have to go the whole distance.

Understanding Natural Cat Behavior

Please refer to Chapter Three, "Cat Scan."

Bonding With Your Cat

Nowadays you frequently hear about the concept of *bonding*. This is a word that's been tossed around for several years, but few really know what it means with respect to pets or how to actually do it.

In human terms bonding is the creation of close, emotional ties with another person. In animal terms it is the pairing between two individual creatures who develop a long-term attachment to each other. That's called *pairbonding*. Through the course of their lives, the two individuals strive never to lose each other.

Bonding can occur between any two people, whether they are husband and wife, parent and child, friends, or lovers. Bonding should also occur between humans and their pets. It is the first necessary step toward successfully living with your cat.

When a cat is secure in the knowledge that he is accepted as a member of the family, he can respond well to any family lifestyle providing he is with those who love him. When the cat is aware of being loved, he feels happy. Being happy becomes a habit and is shared with anyone who comes in contact with that cat. Bonding with your cat brings out the best in both of you.

Is there anything that brings more excitement into your home than the arrival of a new cat, especially a kitten? The anticipation is tantalizing, with daydreams of you and the cat rolling around the carpet after dinner and spending a life of thousands of hugs and games. But the most pleasing day-dream of all is the one where you and the cat become loving friends and develop undying devotion to each other.

These dreams are realities for many cat owners. But they're easy to miss if the cat destroys the new sofa with its claws, constantly scratches your visitors, or causes a lot of arguments between your kids. If your cat is conditioned to behave himself, he is not going to upset you with misbehavior and risk losing your affection. If you understand a few simple rules about cats and children, Tigerboy isn't going to be the cause of dissension in the family. However, everything begins with developing a meaningful relationship, and that involves learning to bond with your new cat.

Bonding with your cat means creating a personal relationship between the two of you with strong feelings of affection. Cats that have bonded with their families usually have a strong desire to be with them. Bonding with your cat not only satisfies your goals concerning him, it paves the way for teaching your cat how to behave himself by making it more pleasant and effective.

Often there is no way to know what your new cat has experienced before he came to live with you. He may have been socialized both to other cats and humans by a knowledgeable breeder and treated well, or his previous life may have been fraught with fear and abuse.

No matter what your kitten's previous life was like, you have an opportunity to communicate to him that he is safe, cherished, and respected. This also applies to a cat who has already been living with you for a while. You can change the relationship with him for the better, even if he is older.

The first thing to do with a new cat is to communicate your affection and not worry about controlling his behavior in any overbearing way. Of course, litter pan orientation should begin the minute the cat comes to live with you. But even here, the underlying philosophy of your cat's education must be that of gentle teaching rather than demanding discipline. Allow your cat to explore his new home, his new world, and to bond with his new family before imposing any aspects of behavior modification. This is especially important if your new cat is a kitten.

The cat's introduction to his home is critical. Everyone in the family should hold him, hug him, and by all means, talk to him. Verbal communication is one of the most important aspects of bonding. It is not foolish to talk to your cat. Naturally, he doesn't understand English, but he does respond to the tone of your voice. Your vocal tone is significant. It conveys all that he needs to know about how you feel about him.

Have you ever watched the parents and friends of a newborn baby? Listen to the ridiculous things they say to the baby, and the way they say them. Then watch the baby's face. The baby may smile or become quiet as he takes in the sounds with wide-eyed fascination. Everything is input to a new baby, and everything you do or say has an influence.

The same is true for a new cat. When you speak to him, the cat listens and then responds. The softer your voice, the sweeter and the higher pitch it is, the more concentrated will be your cat's response to it. The affectionate use of your voice is one of the most important tools you have to help you bond with your cat. It will serve both of you for the rest of your lives together.

Another important way of bonding is touching your cat. One can stroke the cat's fur, pat his head, scratch behind the ears, rub the stomach, and even squeeze the paws. It is always a pleasant surprise for new cat owners when their pets jump onto their laps and ask to be petted. It is the most endearing form of nonverbal communication. Bonding creates warmth and intimacy between cats and humans.

The bonding process helps introduce the cat to his environment and teaches him the routines of his new life. When you're bonding with your cat, it is important to maintain an attitude of teaching without punishments or harsh corrections. Play with your cat often, at different times of the day and evening. Give him several periods of exercise involving tossed toys and rolled balls and ending with small food treats. Develop in the cat's mind his feeding place, his sleeping place, and where he may and may not go. Introducing your cat to his new life and the way you do it is all part of this process. All of these things should be done in a casual, happy manner.

How to play with your cat is an important part of bonding. The right way to play with your cat is in a positive manner that will help the process. Get down on the floor and make yourself available. Play with him, roll over with him, and do the sort of things you would with a crawling baby. This involves play, cuddling, and hugging. Stay away from play that encourages aggressive behavior. Forget tug-of-war and "I've got your nose." You don't want to create a relationship based on bitten fingers and slaps on the face. Remember, if the cat misbehaves, do not holler, hit, or punish him in any way. You wouldn't do that to a baby, and you shouldn't do it to a kitten.

Bonding should involve the entire family, and that includes anyone living under the same roof. Everyone should be encouraged to develop his or her own separate relationship with the cat. The more diverse the relationships the better. The person taking care of the cat's needs is going to have a different kind of bond from the others. She or he will be the nurturing caretaker who feeds the cat, takes him to the vet, and drives him from one place to another. This person will be the substitute mother.

Of course, these responsibilities can be shared, and that is another valid approach to nurturing the cat. For example, a different person can feed the cat each day, or even each meal.

Sharing that responsibility with several people can be good for the cat and the substitute mother. The same holds true for exercising the cat. Playing with the cat can be different in style and manner from one person to another, and that has a positive bonding influence. One person may enjoy throwing a ball for the cat while another person may just like sitting quietly with the cat on his or her lap.

If there are children in the family, one child may choose to relate to the cat as a brother or sister, while another will treat the cat as a close friend. Some adults may even regard the cat as another child. This is a result of personalities, styles, and individual ways of relating to a cat. But cats will accept a relationship on any terms presented without questioning, as long as it is not abusive.

Everyone in the household should bond with the cat in his or her own loving way. It is helpful to ask yourself what kind of bond or relationship you want to have with your cat, because it will be for a lifetime. Always relate to the cat in a way that is comfortable and natural for you. It will help to think of a kitten as a three-month-old baby or a grown cat as an older child. Don't forget, cats are like perpetual preadolescents. They are children that never grow up.

A serious mistake often made by new cat owners and experienced cat owners alike is expecting too much from a cat all at once. A great expectation level can be harmful. New pets and old pets cannot possibly live up to the burden of expectation that is often placed on them. This can create a negative bond or confusion and ambivalence in the cat's mind. It's a lot like raising children in their early years. There are those who try to teach their one- and two-year-olds how to read. As far as one can tell, all that babies can do at that age is see how much food they can drop to the floor from their high chairs. Not much reading is accomplished by one-year-olds.

Here are some activities that help create a strong bond between cats and their families:

- Give the cat a nice name and use it frequently. It is good for him and keeps you in a pleasant frame of mind when relating to him. (If you name your cat Stupid or Barfy, it will be reflected in your manner. There is no way to call a cat Stupid in a nice way.)

Other bonding activities are:

- Determine your cat's personality type (Chapter Two) and respond to it accordingly.
- Feed with affection.
- Talk to your cat with pleasure and excitement.

- Bathe him in a happy, soothing manner.
- Comb and brush him while expressing affection with your hands.
- Introduce the cat to as many new people and different situations as possible.
- Invite the cat to be with you while doing chores.
- Provide frequent play and exercise.
- Implement litter pan training without harshness.
- Provide a consistent daily routine for feeding and playful attention.

Bonding with your cat does not take a very long time. For some it happens in fifteen minutes. For others it may take from one day to one week. However long it takes, it lasts for a lifetime.

Getting Your Cat Under Control

For the specific techniques of cat training see Chapter Six, "How to Train Your Cat."

Creating a good family pet requires getting your cat under control. There are those who will tell you that cat training is unnecessary or impossible to accomplish. Some who should know better refer to training as "cat tricks." Some may even try to convince you that training your cat is ineffective when dealing with problem behavior. Don't you believe it.

Training is just one more way to keep your cat happy. It establishes the boundaries of what your cat is allowed to do and what he is not allowed to do. Your cat depends on you and your family, and if he misbehaves in serious ways, his future with you becomes jeopardized. Training your cat may assure him of keeping his home and a safe place to live.

The essence of cat training is learning how to communicate with your cat. The idea is to communicate what is right and what is wrong. What pleases you and what displeases you.

Cats and the Youngest Members of the Family

Cats and kids are as important a social development as the birthday party. To experienced cat lovers it is no surprise that children adore cats. The trick is to give cats the opportunity to adore children. It would also be valuable for more parents to become aware of the affinity for felines that the youngest members of the family have and to nurture those relationships in a way that enhances the lives of both cats and kids.

The coming together of children and cats is a delightful development, like frozen pudding on a stick or deodorized cat litter. Every child needs a friend who will remain constant and loyal without qualifying the relationship. This kind of friend should not exact a price in exchange for solace and comforting. Where can one turn for such altruistic behavior? To a cat, of course.

Cats are not really psychic, although they certainly have that reputation. All cat owners have at least one wonderful story to tell about their pet coming to them at a dark hour and making life better than it was. What is it that gives cats the superb sense of timing they have when involved in human events? And what is it about cats that creates the magical chemistry that exists between them and children?

Once we get past the false notion that dogs are better for children than cats, it is not too difficult to understand that chemistry. The domestic cat is a vulnerable creature with all of the behavior of a wild animal but only a few of the physical defenses. Consequently, it responds well to gentleness and tender feelings. It does not require ESP for a cat to be attracted to an affectionate, kindly child who has no desire to harm it. If not distorted by harsh influences at home or on the streets, most children have tender feelings toward other living beings and automatically reach out to them. Children have to be taught to dislike snakes or insects, for example. Their natural inclination is to express awe, curiosity, respect, and love. Normal cats like normal children on a direct emotional basis.

It can hardly be a secret that children are intensely interested in animals and all things pertaining to animals. This offers parents the unique opportunity to stimulate learning in their children and, at the same time, exercise significant influence in developing character traits based on important moral codes of behavior. Living with a cat can certainly accomplish this and more. There is no doubt that your cat will help to develop a humane attitude in your child.

Many parents feel that a child begins to learn only when he or she begins school. This is not true. Although parents are the first and most important teachers, children will ever have, house cats can be a strong second.

Most specialists who study child development agree that the first five years are the most formative ones. For cats it is roughly the first year, perhaps the first three months. From infancy on, children try to learn about the world inside and outside the home as well as the feelings inside themselves, such as happiness, sadness, anger, fear, and frustration. They want to manipulate, investigate, imitate, and master as much of their environment as they can. To children, learning is a natural and joyful experience. The same is true of kittens. Together, cats and kids can grow stronger, healthier, and more vital.

A responsive and accepting relationship between a child and a pet helps to enhance a sense of belonging in the child, a sense of responsibility to him- or herself and to others, and the ability to learn and make decisions. These first attitudes will certainly have an influence throughout the life of the child. There are no hard and fast rules for developing the relationship between a child and a cat. Different approaches are necessary between individual children and their cats because of the varied lifestyles of families as they exist nowadays. However, one can examine existing, general guidelines to help develop happy, self-confident, and self-disciplined children who just happen to treat their cats well.

Self-Image

The way a child learns to handle and care for a cat helps in developing a healthy self-image. When children like themselves, they believe they are worthwhile people. When children do not have a sound and healthy self-image, if they do not like themselves or if they believe others do not like them, they tend to show it by being aggressive or withdrawn. They may hurt others in order to ease their own inner pain or avoid thinking something that they consider unacceptable. They may also withdraw into a shell, a personal and private world, to protect themselves from what they believe is rejection. Obviously, the primary source of self-esteem is one's parents. But do not discount the value of living with a cat.

If you help a child set realistic goals with regard to caring for a cat, your child is more apt to experience the elated feeling of achievement and success. This in turn allows for feelings of competence in dealing with life problems as they are encountered. For example, learning the proper way to hold a cat without dropping the animal is good for a child's self-image. The approved method is to slip one hand under the cat's chest, holding the front legs gently but firmly with the fingers, while at the same time, cupping the other hand under the cat's hindquarters. Do not pick up a cat by the scruff of the neck. Never allow a child to grab the cat by the forelegs or place an arm around the stomach.

But what if your child is simply too young or not strong enough to do this. Then ask the child to help you hold the cat but you do the lifting. That is acceptable. Offer congratulations for helping you properly and tell the child that soon she or he will be able to handle the cat alone. This is realistic without a built-in failure . . . and, to be sure, will be easier on the cat.

It is also rewarding to encourage the child to express thoughts, feelings, and ideas concerning the cat. Allow the child to shop for the cat's needs, participate in the decision-making process (e.g. food selection, toys, bedding, and so on). It is quite reassuring for the child to discover that she or he has an important role in the family, that the family cares about how the child feels and what the child thinks, says, and does.

The basic attitudes that make up self-image develop out of what is learned from those who love the child and whom the child loves best. Although this applies most importantly to the family, the cat can be a vital element here. The emotional exchange between a youngster and a cat and the lessons a cat teaches about behavior is of enormous value. Children soon discover that cats respond best to gentle, kind treatment. They also learn that aggressive, abusive behavior earns them the same in kind plus personal rejection. Rejection from a cat is a natural consequence of shabby treatment of the cat. This is a self-correcting feature built into the relationship. Dealing well with the world outside of the home is an outgrowth of dealing well within it. One's self-image plays a major role.

Responsibility

When children are three, four, and five years of age, they often delight in proving how grown-up they are. Giving children small responsibilities in the home makes them feel needed and helps them become competent as well as self-confident. Applying this idea to cat care is a sound idea. Some parents, however, go overboard, especially with older children, and simply set the scene for failure by demanding too much. There are some aspects of cat care that should always be handled by an adult. However, many activities connected with the cat's health and happiness can and should be the sole province of the younger members of the household. It all depends on the child's age, desire, and abilities. Arrange for your child to be successful in the early stages of the task he or she is learning. Start with simple jobs and work up to more difficult ones as skills increase. Design or alter the activity according to her or his level of development. Suit the tasks to the child's individual interests. It is important to be cheerful, supportive, and understanding when the child's capability or interest diminishes. Show your willingness to be helpful. The child who is given help when needed is best prepared to give help to others when they need it.

Feeding the cat. This is one job that a child can handle with ease and pleasure. Toddlers can at least get out the food and hand it to you. For a very young child it is a satisfying accomplishment. Cleaning food and water bowls can be handled, in part, by children of almost any age and the same applies to the cleaning of the cat's living areas. Most young children like to sweep and work the vacuum cleaner.

Grooming the cat. This is an especially useful activity. Daily grooming is a necessary chore and can provide a pleasant time for both child and cat. The most important aspect of grooming is combing and brushing the animal's fur. This must be accomplished every day not only for the sake of a good appearance but to avoid the ill effects of the animal's constant licking of its own coat. Daily brushing and combing makes the animal look and feel better and helps to avoid hair balls from developing in the stomach. If a kitten is combed and brushed daily, it is less likely to fight grooming later on as many cats do.

Combing or brushing out a cat requires physical contact, and that in turn deepens the relationship between animal and human. It is a loving gesture that cannot be mistaken for anything else. For our purposes, loving contact is much more important than whether or not the coat looks perfect.

When a child handles a brush or comb, it must be applied to the cat very gently and slowly. Teach your child to speak soothingly as she or he grooms, so that the entire experience is one that the cat will look forward to. Some grown cats hate being groomed, and some change their minds about it after years of acceptance. Do not take it as a personal rejection if your cat does not allow himself to be groomed. Learn how to groom from a professional groomer or from a book.

The best brushes are made of natural bristles and do not irritate the skin or pull the hair. A small hard-rubber brush is useful for short-coated cats. A half-fine/half-medium stainless steel comb with tapered teeth is the best and most versatile to own. The length of the teeth determine if it is suitable for a long- or short-coated cat. The teeth of the comb must be long enough to reach down through the coat to the skin. Whether or not to bathe your cat is a personal decision based on your child, your cat, and your stomach lining.

When assigning your child cat-care responsibilities ask

yourself the following questions: Is it a job he can do well? Is there enough time to accomplish the task? Did she help decide if she wanted to do that particular job? Is it very important to the cat? To the family? Is it too routine and boring? Are you giving enough praise and recognition for a job well done? Are you taking for granted a good performance while criticizing poor performance? Does the child feel good about doing the job? The answers to these questions can tell you if you are being reasonable and explain any discontentment in the child.

Play Time

In addition to aiding emotional and psychological growth, cats also perform another large service for children. They provide a great degree of stimulation and fun. Perhaps that is the most wonderful part of cats and kids. For the most part a cat and a child play well together. If you visit a good nursery school or kindergarten, you will quickly discover that play is the principal activity. However, if you look more carefully you will also discover that the play is carefully orchestrated. Although there are many periods of free play, most of the time is spent in playlike activities. The reason for this is that professional teachers and child experts understand that play is a learning experience. It teaches through the process of repetition, reenactment, emulation, and, of course, instruction.

Kittens, grown cats, and children of all ages have a great desire and need to play. It is built into our systems. That is how we learn; how we release our energies and tensions; how we relieve boredom and frustration. Play is a form of recreation, which actually means to refresh the mind and body, to re-create ourselves. Play can be a regeneration of the spirit as well as a teaching process.

Kittens learn how to survive in a wild state (that they almost never experience) through the various forms of play activity. Adult cats never seem to lose the desire for these survival games, nor do other species of cat. Cat play seems to reduce itself to stalking, pouncing, prey capture, and fighting. These play activities are carried out, usually, with more exuberance than the circumstances require. When kittens play, they scratch and bite, but not seriously.

The play behavior of children is often a recreation of adult situations and responses to those situations. You can probably find out much more about your neighbors, if that is what interests you, by watching and listening to their children at play. What is important to understand is that play behavior is species specific. What is play for cats is not necessarily play for humans. However, the spirit of play is very similar, and this is where children and cats are at their best. To a child, as to a cat, play should be exuberant and fun, always fun.

The use of balls, spools of thread, and all manner of things that roll simulates the movement of prey animals to a cat. If you roll a Ping-Pong ball across the floor, a kitten will probably wait for it to stop, stalk it, pounce upon it, and then wrestle with it. A litter of kittens or several grown cats will tussle and roll over one another one minute as if engaged in a life-or-death struggle and then the next minute lick and groom one another. Dangle a string and it becomes a flying insect. Flutter a peacock feather and it becomes a bird to capture. Give a cat a paper bag and watch it become a cave or an intruder to fight with. Place a walnut in an empty tissue box and watch it transform into a hiding mouse. Sock toys, shoe boxes, cardboard cartons, yarn, feather dusters, and so on, provide wonderful opportunities for play between cats and kids. All you really have to do is prime the imagination with ideas about hunting, tigers, jungles, mountains, and all manner of things pertaining to cats and their wilder cousins. A cat can also become a make-believe person to a child. The key to play is the word "pretend."

Solace

During the course of childhood there are many transitional periods of growth and development. Each new phase is fraught with fear of the new way of being and a refusal to give up the old way. Trading off the security of dependency for the unknown factors of independence creates stormy emotions and a deeply felt ambivalence. This is true for every child.

Cats respond sympathetically and most lovingly to the somber moods of children. It is a lucky child that has a pet cat during those times when life is difficult and the world does not seem to be a happy place. When a child is confused and troubled, her or his cat will always be there to offer a bit of warmth and friendship, consistency, and unquestioned loyalty. That's a lot better than retrieving a thrown stick.

Cats Are Good for Kids and Vice-Versa

We are told that cats are not really good for children, especially young children; they are too self-centered to relate to an outgoing child. We are told that kids are no good for cats; they are too harmful, destructive, and insensitive. We are told that children are too rough-and-tumble for the fragile, delicate physique of cats; that the animals will suffer with twisted tails or broken bones. Some spoilers indicate that cats cause harm to children by slashing them with claws as they slather. To those who are conversant with kids and cats, this is pure kitty litter. Most cats, especially those that have been socialized at an early age, are gentle, loving creatures that want little more than to be fed on time and given a soft lap to sit on.

Do no harm. Cats almost never harm children. When they do, it is the exception rather than the rule. A cat starts out neutral. How a child relates to the cat determines the outcome. A hardback edition of Mother Goose can be an uplifting, educational experience for a child, or it can be used by one child to bop another on the head. Normal, healthy cats will respond sweetly to good care, gentle treatment, affection, and companionship. But all creatures must be permitted to respond in terms that are unique to their natures.

There are only three potential hazards when mixing cats and kids:

1. Diseases transmitted by animals
2. Allergies
3. Injury due to bites and scratches.

Disease. A few simple guidelines help avoid the possibility of household pets transmitting disease to humans. With care, family pets probably offer little or no health hazard to young children. First and most obvious, keep pets healthy by having them checked by a veterinarian at least once a year, maintaining their immunization annually, and having them checked for worms once or twice a year.

Sick animals should be separated from the family. If the illness is more than minor or persists beyond two or three days, the animal should be examined and treated by a veterinarian. If the disease is considered transmissible to humans, advice should be sought from a physician.

Cats can acquire and then transmit several common diseases, including ringworm, tapeworm, salmonella, and various fungal, bacterial, and viral infections. It is wise to separate cats infected with diseases that are transmissible to humans from children and other members of the family.

Animals should be kept clean and free of parasites such as fleas and ticks. They should be bathed periodically and the areas where they sleep and play kept clean.

Allergies. It is difficult to predict whether a given individual will demonstrate an allergy to a specific animal or pet without protracted medical tests administered by an allergist. If there is a history of allergies in your family, it is possible for your child to be more susceptible to allergens from animals. However, many children from such families never experience difficulties from house pets. Look for respiratory or dermatological symptoms. These indicate the need for medical attention.

Injuries. When children and pets are brought together, care and supervision is necessary for the good of both. Some cats, particularly older ones, do not tolerate the unpredictable behavior of young children. Rarely, if ever, will they deliberately attack a child, but if teased, tormented or cornered they may lash out.

Cats and New Babies

Cats often have noticeable emotional responses when a new baby appears in the family. This behavior has been described as sibling rivalry or jealousy, with the pet demanding more attention than usual or perhaps ignoring the owners or refusing to eat. Often the cat expresses his unhappiness by developing temporary housebreaking difficulties. Cats rarely become upset enough to cause harm to a new baby. The opposite reaction is the normal one, with the family pet devoting full time to guarding the baby or at least staring at it with awe.

It is essential to allow the cat a period of adjustment when a new baby is brought into the family. The pet may need extra attention and should never be left alone with the baby. In general, with reasonable care, a cat is not a health hazard to a new baby. Clearly it is an added responsibility for parents, but the enjoyment and advantages provided by the cat far outweigh the added burden.

When a new baby is brought into the home, the cat should be invited to inspect the new addition to the family. At first, the animal may be a bit hesitant (many babies are bigger than cats). After an hour or two the cat may approach the baby, give it a few perfunctory sniffs, and walk away. By evening, things are sure to be normal, and the cat will resume enjoying his life, including hopping onto a motherly lap (shared with an infant).

Children ranging from one to four years of age, and many older ones too, enjoy cats more than dogs if the cats are even the least bit friendly. When infants and toddlers are properly guided when touching a cat, they express joy from the sensuous pleasure of stroking the animal's luxurious fur. Most cats will sit still (at least for a minute) and enjoy the gentle fondling and added attention from the youngest member of the family.

Babies smile with surprise and delight when a cat meows or hunches its body to stretch. Cats do not overwhelm them with boundless energy as a dog will. Another dividend: A docile cat affords a toddler the opportunity to share a private world that no adult can intrude upon, and that's a wonderful gift to give any child.

There are some practical considerations for cat owners, though, if they have small children—especially infants. A cat's nails should be clipped often. An infant or small child should never be left alone with a cat (or a dog), and the child should be taught by example and direct instruction how to pet and touch the animal. (The hand should be flat and glide across the animal with ease in a loving, caressing manner, gently stroking with the lay of the fur.)

This is no small matter. It is the beginning of humane behavior and attitudes that affect the child for a lifetime.

Helping children develop an ethical system in which kindness to animals is regarded as essential is important business. It is doubtful that one who abuses animals can be sensitive toward people. The mental and spiritual health of children can be greatly influenced for the good by teaching the value of kindness and respect for all living creatures. A child who has been taught to hold, caress, and cherish a loving cat knows more about survival and sanity than a stadium full of world leaders and politicians.

Pets are good friends but also members of the family. Acquiring a pet may be the only opportunity a child will ever have to choose a relative. The pet connection could easily become the most valuable experience your child will have short of school and four years with an orthodontist. That is why it is a good thing for parents to allow their kids the wonderful involvement with a cat.

Schedule for Children's Cat-Care Responsibilities

Toddlerhood

This period lasts from approximately nine months to three years. So much is happening in a child's development during these months that one would hardly think cat-care responsibilities are appropriate. Not true. There are some cat-connected activities that provide an ideal outlet for a toddler's boundless curiosity and desire to discover the world. There are no cat chores for a child of this age that can be competently achieved without a parent's assistance, but the rewards for allowing the toddler to participate in the family cat's activities are very great. Self-sufficiency, creative play, a sense of individuality, feelings of competency, being a part of the family are just some of the benefits derived by a toddler who helps her or his parents or brothers and sisters take care of their cat.

When a toddler is past eighteen months, she or he is able to help empty the grocery bag and carry the cat's food from the bag to the table. The same applies to the shelf on which it's stored. The simple act of handing you the can or box of cat food may not seem like much, but is certain to make your child feel truly accomplished.

At two years old a child can help you with other tasks connected with the cat. For example, when you wash the cat's food and water bowls, your assistant can attempt to dry them (if you show how). It would be a good idea to check the work and point out the moisture the child didn't get. Once the bowls are completely dry, both you and the toddler can pour or spoon the cat food and water into them. Caution: Do not allow a toddler to hand the food to the cat or get too close to the feeding area on the floor. Some cats misinterpret the child's presence at their food and become aggressive. To avoid the possibility of getting bitten, the child should never get too close to the cat while he is being fed or actually eating. It could make him snap or bite. It can be dangerous with some cats.

A two-year-old can also help a parent tidy up the cat's area, be it a cat bed, or a corner of the kitchen with a pillow on the floor. Minor tasks involving a cleaning cloth or whisk broom are ideal. You might even give your toddler a turn with the mop. At this age many children love to help out with chores as a way of testing their competency by imitating their parents. It is a rare opportunity to develop in the child the pleasure and gratification of responsibility.

From nine months to three years, children understand so much more than adults realize. This may be because of their limited use of speech. Their powers of comprehension far exceed their desire or ability to use language actively. If you speak slowly and simply, at eye level, a toddler will understand what it is you want him or her to do. Once the request is made, it is up to the parent to take the child by the hand and begin the assignment. Remember, the child is only assisting you and must be instructed and supervised. Once the task has been completed (or seems so to the child), inspect the work and offer your praise and congratulations. Tell the cat what a good job your little girl or boy has done and elicit some enthusiasm from the pet. Cats get excited when their owners get excited. They quickly perceive human emotions and get caught up in them. It is therefore not difficult to make the cat appear to praise your toddler for a job well done.

Three to Five

Children of this age group may help prepare the cat's meals (although they should not feed the animal directly). They may continue to help clean the cat's utensils, living areas, and house areas where the cat has shed fur or knocked things over. During this period most children develop a greater attention span and are capable of more difficult tasks. They are more self-confident and able to exercise greater patience. Their language has become fluid and understandable. Children between three and five can take a more responsible position for the cat. This sense of responsibility is highly desirable because of the cat's difficulty later in accepting status changes in members of his family.

Three- to five-year-old children stand well above the average-sized cat. This is not necessarily threatening to the cat, providing the child's behavior does not indicate a challenge to his position of dominance. Let us not forget that for three years (one-sixth of the average cat's lifetime) the family pet has viewed the young child from infancy to toddlerhood as a kitten or subordinate member of the family. If the cat has always taken a leader's position in the family, then there may be trouble ahead for a growing child. Even a cat that has been subordinate to other members of the family may feel threatened by the transition of a child's size and behavior as the years pass.

Although it has not been ascertained scientifically, it is safe to assume that there is a time in the family cat's life when he accepts the fluctuations of family structure and resigns himself to the idea that there is one less subordinate member in his family. Prior to acceptance, there may be a defensive-aggressive action resulting in a young child's getting bitten. There is no reason why parents cannot prevent this type of incident if they intelligently shape the relationship between cat and child. It is during this period of childhood (three to five) that the preventive measures can be taken.

A child in this age range is still learning from parental example. Therefore his or her parents must relate to the cat in a loving but firm tone of voice when giving him instructions. The child can be guided to relate in the same manner. Everything must be done to encourage the child to take a leadership position in relationship to the cat, but it must be done gently and as smoothly as possible. Anything that places the child in a responsible position over the cat is desirable, providing the parent is there to prevent the cat from rebelling. Remember: A three- to five-year-old is too immature in manner and physical presence to truly take care of the average adult cat.

Take things slowly, without expecting too much of the child or the cat. This is merely the beginning of a slow transition in their relationship. It is very encouraging to note that most cats adore their young family members once they are able to spend time together without adult supervision. That comes later. But a cat and an older child hanging out together is a joyous sight. This is the time to prepare for that.

Six to Ten

There seems to be general agreement among child experts that the age of six is a difficult one for many children. Six is an age of emotional extremes. The child's a confusing mixture of baby and child, and parents often find him or her quite difficult to handle.

This is a time when a child is breaking away from total dependency on the home and parents and is forcing himself or herself to explore the world outside. It is also the time when most children begin formal schooling, which can be an emotional drain. It is probably not a good time to make very many demands in regard to cat care. A six-year-old can be obstinate, easily distracted, and insistent on doing things his or her own way (whether right or wrong). However, the need for a cat's love may be greater than ever. It is probably best to allow a child of six to accept whatever responsibilities he or she can handle for the cat and not push things too far. For the sake of the cat's needs, other members of the family should assume full responsibility for the animal's care until this difficult period is over.

Seven to ten is quite another matter when it comes to cat care. At this age there are few chores connected with a cat that a child cannot accomplish. Still, you must supervise and, at times, assist in various activities, such as grooming, baths, medical treatment. A young child in this age range should not have to take a pet to the veterinarian's office unescorted. It's a good idea for a young cat owner to share that responsibility with a parent. It is a question of the seriousness of the cat's illness in relationship to the degree of sensitivity of the child to such situations. If a cat is extremely sick or near death, it may be a good idea to allow the child to witness those events and procedures leading to euthanasia or natural death. Bearing witness to the truth is a good rule to live by and applies to the unhappy aspects of life as well as any other. It is, of course, a matter of parental discretion.

An eight-, nine-, or ten-year old is old enough and strong enough to deal with a pet cat's elimination needs. Indoor cats, of course, use a litter pan, and it must be kept in a clean, sanitary condition. A clean litter pan is not only for the humans' sensibilities but for the cat's as well. The issue for the cat is not hygiene alone. Few cats will use a litter pan that has not been cleaned out frequently. It will cause them to find a new place to eliminate on, usually the floor in a corner of the room. Have your ten-year-old scoop the litter pan once or even twice a day and change the sand or other material once or twice a week.

Children between the ages of six and ten may now participate in feeding the family pet but must be gentle and not make too much of a fuss when presenting the dish. Some cats become used to one person, usually an adult, feeding them and may refuse to eat if the food is handled by a younger member of the family. In the natural state cats hunt alone for their food and eat it by themselves. They are always vulnerable to a larger animal stealing it. A domestic cat has inherited a somewhat suspicious nature and does not trust anyone coming near his food. Unless the family cat has come to accept a child as the one who provides his meals, he is going to be uneasy about that child being near his food. It takes a while for the cat to understand that the child is not taking, but rather giving, the food. It helps if you are present as the child feeds the cat. Ideally, both parent and child together should position the food in its proper place. This helps the cat to accept the child fully.

Another responsibility for children of this age is the cat's need for exercise. There is probably no greater exercise for a cat than a good romping play period with children. Every house or apartment offers its own set of physical limitations on this kind of play. But there is always room enough for some degree of physical play between a child and a cat, and it is such a desirable activity that it is well worth the noise and inconvenience. Here is a responsibility that every child will enjoy and benefit from at the same time. Both cat and child are not only exercised but enjoy the development of strong bonds of friendship as they interact. They will play, and then they will relax and enjoy each other's company in a way that few adults can experience. A Ping-Pong ball, a stick with a string at the end, or a cardboard box or paper bag is almost all that is needed for this purpose. Of course the child must be guided so that the cat is not hurt or overstimulated. Some cats really want to call it quits but the child continues, unaware of the animal's exhaustion or oncoming irritability. This problem is easily solved by parents setting a time limit on the play-exercise period and also by confining it to one room.

Eleven and Twelve

This stage of childhood is referred to as preadolescence. Many physical and mental developments are taking place at the same time, and they often conflict with one another, as when the dependencies of childhood clash with the drive toward independence. Large, overpowering emotions can erupt from eleven- and twelve-year-olds. Sometimes those feelings are not fully expressed but just seething under the surface. Emotions range from one extreme to another, and one can see joy and despair, elation and dejection from day to day, or sometimes from hour to hour. Children of this age are often moody, suspicious, or irritable. Because this is in part a difficult period for adult and child alike, the pleasures of cat ownership can be especially beneficial. Being totally responsible for the needs and desires of a cat offers the immeasurable reward of self-confidence and gives your child an understanding of his or her competence. With the exception of the cat's medical needs (veterinary examinations, home nursing procedures, and home diagnoses) and, to some extent, cat training, an eleven- or twelve-year-old child can assume all responsibilities for a cat.

The right cat with the right child can offer the ideal private relationship that does not have to be shared. With luck and parental skill, an eleven- or twelve-year-old might just find in a cat the middle ground between emotional turmoil and family love. It is important here to consider the well-being of the cat. Therefore it must be made clear that with the comfort the cat brings must also come a dedication to its care. If the child cannot enter into such an agreement, it is best for all concerned to forgo the relationship and allow the animal to become the family pet. However, it is difficult to imagine a cat not being able to burrow beneath the barriers of preadolescence and relate lovingly to any child.

Thirteen to Fifteen

Probably the most important liberty for the early teenage child is the freedom of choice. Finding out what your teenager prefers and allowing for independent decisions in regard to cat ownership is essential. Allow for the inconsistencies between declarations of independence and quiet requests for money and other kinds of assistance. Once your teenager takes on the burden of cat care, don't be surprised if a little neglect or abdication of some responsibilities creeps in along the edges. Discussions and adjustments of cat-care responsibilities will probably be in order. The many benefits of a relationship between a human and a cat have all been stated before and apply to a greater degree with a teenager.

A girl or a boy between thirteen and fifteen years old can take on any and all aspects of cat care providing the teenager understands that the cat's very life is in his or her hands. Probably the most worthwhile and rewarding responsibility for a child in this age range is training the cat. There is much to be learned through this activity, by cat and child. With the help of training instructions such as those provided in Chapter Six, "How to Train Your Cat," both cat and child learn to bring order to confusion and chaos. For the cat, there is the security of affirming his position in the family. For the child, cat training offers lessons in leadership, self-discipline, and the performance of social responsibilities.

5

A CAT AND
A DOG

A dog and cat sharing the same home is like a vaudevillian horse. It's hard to tell who's in front and who's in back until the performers come out of the equine suit to take a bow. However, the most significant aspect of the situation is that necessity has made both partners inseparable. There is a popular misconception that dogs rule the roost and cats tread lightly around the old doghouse. Those who believe that have been watching too many cartoons. Our pussyfooted friends are not necessarily the submissive quadrupeds we think they are. Dogs know it, and it's time that everybody else knows it too. Although dogs and cats sharing the same home develop meaningful relationships, till death do they part, they do it in species-specific ways.

Surveys tell us that millions of American families live with one or more dogs and one or more cats together in the same home. Contrary to popular mythology dogs and cats can, for the most part, live quite well together, sharing territory, food, and human contact. Human attitudes toward pet dogs and cats lie somewhere between Saturday morning cartoons and comic books, which hardly offer a realistic view of dog and cat behavior.

The saving grace is the dynamic interaction between four-legged and two-legged creatures. The human desire to live with dogs and cats seems to be connected with avoiding human overpopulation. Even more significant is dog and cat acceptance and (in many cases) the pleasure of sharing a mutual existence. One could argue that a canine and feline have no choice once thrown together and therefore must find a way to make it work. To some degree this is true. However, anyone living in this human/animal configuration knows there is more to it than simple accommodation. Dogs and cats often develop the most poignant relationships and share a world together that is as meaningful as that of any two humans.

Keeping dogs and cats in one home may or may not be a natural check-and-balance technique for limiting the human population by having pets instead of babies. It is a debatable argument. Whatever has caused this cultural-biological-ethological phenomenon is beside the point. The significant aspect of living with dogs and cats together is that it's an enjoyable and civilizing experience. It is also a fascinating experiment in nature. When two totally different kinds of animals are thrown together and make their adjustments so that survival is assured and the fulfillment of animal destiny is realized, it can be a fascinating experience.

In one such situation a kitten was acquired as a companion for a six-month-old Siberian husky puppy. Huskies cannot bear to be alone for even one hour. When left alone this particular young dog howled and warbled, disturbing the neighbors. The kitten was brought in to alleviate the dog's feeling of aloneness. He solved the problem. At first the young cat arched his back and hissed his full eight weeks' worth of fury at the sight of the gangly young dog. The husky jumped around energetically, sending the kitten scampering under the couch. Despite this unpromising beginning the two animals developed a close relationship and came to depend on each other. They were inseparable.

The pressure was definitely off the human family as the dog and cat amused each other with wrestling, running, and jumping all over the place. When the dog was taken out for a walk, the cat paced back and forth at the front door in anticipation of the dog's return. Over the years they developed games they both played and enjoyed and they shared a very peaceable kingdom. As their family started having children, the dog and cat became even closer to each other, replacing the attention they had lost. In the beginning the kitten was very much under the domination of the dog, which must be attributed to the disparity of size and maturity. The dog was three months older than the cat and in their first year together was significantly larger and more behaviorally developed. As they entered their second year together their relationship began to change. What seemed to be greater tolerance of the cat's behavior by the dog was in reality the cat coming into his own as an adult male of his species.

The behavior of cats and dogs is quite different, but their differences are not based on one being a more dominant animal than the other. Quite the contrary. They are both species that develop a dominant/subordinate order within the societies of their respective species. As stated earlier, dog behavior is similar to wolf behavior. Pack structure is the most important aspect of wild behavior for the average dog owner to understand. Wolves most often live and thrive in packs or loose-knit families consisting of close relatives, distant relatives, and occasional nonrelated individuals. They are led by a dominant male who is usually the most aggressive wolf in the pack. The pack itself develops a social order of rank based on dominance and submission. This too is of vital importance to dog owners. Domestic dogs, like wolves, develop social attachments based on an order of rank and for the most part adhere to it rigidly, except on those rare occasions when the pack leader is challenged.

This social lifestyle is genetically organized into their behavior. Therefore, when a dog is taken to its new home, the human family substitutes for the more natural pack. This is true even if the family consists of one human and one or two other companion animals. From the dog's perspective the territory belonging to the pack (or human family) is the apartment or house, with or without acreage. That is why dogs take to family life so naturally. A young dog, even an aggressive one, will quickly sort out in his mind who is dominant and who isn't within the pack structure of the human family (and that includes cats as well).

Cats are not animals oriented to a social order, at least not one that we commonly recognize. Most wild cats are solitary creatures who come together for mating and rearing their young. At all other times both males and females live separately within their exclusive ranges and territories, with the exception of lions who live in prides (a kind of pack). This solitary lifestyle in the wild is the foreshadowing behavior of most domestic cats. It is why they appear to be independent and often indifferent to human pampering. Over the generations of domestic pampering humans have treated their pet cats like children or, more significantly, like kittens. This has encouraged cats to behave in an infantile or adolescent manner. Thus we have a feline creature that wants to be fed on schedule, groomed, played with, and given parental affection. How unlike their image, not to mention their wild "grown-up" cousins.

When one witnesses two or more cats living together and getting along, it is because they are adhering to an instinct to sort themselves out in some social order of top cat and low cat. However, in cat societies that can change suddenly and even frequently. It is based on the behavior of shifting social rank in an uncontrolled mating situation that can be witnessed in any backyard.

What domestic dogs and domestic cats have in common is a dependency created by human indulgence and kindness. Emotional and physical dependency created by humans is what allows dogs and cats to live together sharing the same home, the same human caretakers. Although dogs and cats are not natural enemies, neither are they natural friends. They too often compete for space, food, water, human contact, and attention.

Male dogs (and some females) that are highly territorial, especially among the terriers, the working breeds, and some of the sporting breeds, are very dominant in nature and quite assertive. However, some cats are also dominant in their behavior. A dominant dog stakes out specific objects and locations as territorial boundaries and can get quite ugly about them. Most common of these are food and water bowls, sleeping quarters, a special corner of a room, and even a person. Although some cats also prize these objects and locations, they will rarely fight over them, unless it's with another cat. Cats become more assertive about pathways leading to favored locations, attention from favored individuals, food treats not on the daily menu, play objects, catnip, and sex objects.

In most dog-cat households the two animals rarely want what's important to the other, and that's what makes it all work. Unfortunately, that is not always the case. Many a dog has received an embedded cat claw in his nose because he went that extra step. There can be no doubt that a large, aggressive dog will gain the upper hand over a cat, providing the cat is caught off guard. But heaven help a dog that backs a mature cat into a corner in a threatening way. In the end, the dog may win out, but he will have paid a terrible physical price. This rarely happens, because in the early stages of a dog-cat relationship one takes full measure of the other and behaves with common sense. Over the years the two animals will sort things out, for the most part, and learn to stay away from each other's sensitive areas.

The most successful dog-cat relationships are developed when the animals are introduced to each other as puppies and kittens. However, a very young kitten will imprint on a grown dog with greater ease than a puppy or young dog on a grown cat. Because there are so many variables, one must allow for many exceptions to the rule. An old cat can make an adjustment to a new dog under the right circumstances, although it is difficult. Because of an adolescent dog's desire to play and romp, it will try to draw an older cat into dozens of daily games and add new vitality to the cat's life. It can make the older animal feel somewhat like a kitten again.

Dogs and cats have needs that sometimes blend and sometimes clash at different periods of their lives and create the shifting sands of dominance and submission. A teething dog or a cat in heat should be separated from the other animal until one or the other is behaving normally.

Terriers and some hunting dogs should not be allowed near newborn kittens as they are apt to mistake them for rodents and harm them. Some dogs who are avowed cat haters will develop a loving relationship with the family cat while hating them as a species and continuing to attack strays that wander into their territory. An assertive unaltered male cat would not have the subordinate manner necessary to get along with a large, territorial dog.

The conduct of the human family often determines what the relationship between a cat and dog will be like. Here are some guidelines:

1. If possible, bring a dog and cat together when they are young. The most successful dog-cat relationships are developed when the animals are introduced as puppies and kittens. However, a young kitten will attach itself to a grown dog and develop a subordinate relationship to it. Introducing a puppy to a grown cat is more difficult and requires a lot more time, patience, and supervision.

2. Establish a well-defined dog-cat system within your house. Give each animal an area exclusively his own. Place their *dens* or *lairs* as far apart as possible and at different heights. For a dog, a carton with a blanket placed in the corner of a room or basement is sufficient, although a wire dog crate is best.

Some cats prefer soft, pillowlike beds and baskets designed just for them, while others enjoy a simple cardboard box. If possible, give the cat a territory on a level higher than the dog's, such as a food bowl on a table or mantel. Place the cat's bed on the second floor or on a table. The ideal resting place for a cat is a tall "cat tree," which is something like a pole with carpeted platforms placed on it at various heights. These are sold in pet supply catalogs and at cat shows. Advertisements for such cat furniture are seen in all cat magazines.

3. Feed your pets at different times and in different places. Special attention such as baths and other grooming procedures should be given when the other pet is not present.

4. Obedient pets are more likely to live in harmony with each other than those without organized behavioral responses to human commands. Train your dog and cat. You can have a dog trained by a professional in your home, attend an obedience training class, or you can do it yourself with the help of a dog training book. A cat is usually trained by its owner. See Chapter Six, "How to Train Your Cat."

5. Pay attention to each animal's needs. At times these need blend and at times they clash. If the dog or cat, for instance, becomes sick, they should be separated from each other because a sick animal is often not friendly to anyone. As stated earlier, some dogs mistake newborn kittens for prey animals and attack them. Never allow a dog to come near a litter of kittens, as it upsets the mother even if the dog is merely curious.

Most dogs and cats get along with each other, and in many cases actually develop important, meaningful relationships. Depending on temperament, early socialization, obedience training, and a loving environment, most dogs will adjust to the most impudent of cats and most cats will make peace with the most assertive dogs. It is all influenced by human behavior. The first multi-pet household was the Ark and that worked out pretty well.

6

HOW TO TRAIN
YOUR CAT

Of course cats can be trained, but it's a walk on the wild side. Rarely do they hand you their paw, roll over and play dead, or jump through a hoop on command (unless it was their own idea). Training cats has limitations. They will allow themselves to be taught a few things if there is some advantage for them, such as food rewards. Cats are intelligent creatures with a marvelous problem-solving ability, but most training must coincide with their natural inclinations. Cats only appear to be stubborn. Their behavior is mostly predetermined by instinct, inherited family traits, and early influences, leaving only a little ability for adapting to new conditions and inducements.

Dogs, on the other hand, are social animals and are more than willing to please in exchange for human approval. Cats are not at all like that. House cats become attached to humans when treated with care and affection and return their affection only when it is not demanded of them. If you combined a highly qualified love with various dependencies, you'd have the emotional life of the domestic cat. Cats are independent because of their instinctive solitary lifestyle and their ability to resort to predatory skills if forced to live on their own in the wild state. However, house cats living as pets need humans to feed them, clean their litter

145

boxes, let them in and out, supply the catnip, and protect them from galloping dogs and clutchy children. It is within these domestic needs that cat training becomes possible.

Contrary to popular belief, most cats can be trained to some degree and, indeed, must be trained if they are going to share the human environment. Cats must be taught to use their litter pans or the outdoors for their toileting. They should be taught to come to you when you call them; to walk with you on a leash; to sit when you tell them; and to respond to the human demand "No!"

There are several factors that determine a cat's ability to be trained. If he has remained with his mother for the first eight weeks of life, he has been taught certain fundamentals. One of the most important lessons learned is the idea of burying urine and feces so its presence cannot be detected by enemies or prey animals. One can clearly see the relationship between this behavior and learning to use a litter pan. It becomes natural and logical for a kitten entering a new home. He need only be shown where the pan is and be placed inside. Finding and capturing prey are also taught by the mother. Fighting, escape behavior, and prey capture techniques are learned mostly through play behavior during the rough-and-tumble encounters between kittens of the same litter.

The most important factor in a cat's ability to be educated is his opportunity to be socialized. In the earliest weeks of his life, a kitten should be handled and cuddled by a human several times a day. He should also be surrounded by objects such as toys, spools, balls, and yarn to stimulate mental and physical activity. If these elements are introduced early in a kitten's life, he will be much more adaptive to living with and responding to human beings as well as other cats. A socialized cat will respond to training more enthusiastically. It is almost never too late to socialize an older cat to some degree of adaptability. Although kittens should stay with their mothers until weaned (eight to ten weeks), loving human contact is essential as soon as possible. Some researchers and breeders believe this contact may be started from the first day of life.

Positive Inducement

Unlike dogs, cats must be convinced that learning something new is to their advantage. Positive inducement (bribery) is the key element in most cat training, unless you're dealing with negative behavior such as scratching or chewing plants.

What works for training cats is that they are locked into their own predictable behavior patterns and minor vices. By knowing what pleases your cat, you can develop his responses to your commands through food and affection bribery. If you smear a little butter on his paws, he can be distracted from anything; a commercial cat snack will certainly get his attention; give him a cheese omelet and he'll follow you anywhere.

An effective teaching inducement is a reward of yeast tablets which can be obtained at a health food store. Most cats adore them, and they are quite healthful when given in moderation. One or two at a time is about the correct amount to feed during any training session. A high-quality catnip also makes a good training reward, but should not be given until after the session is over. Some cats take a while to recover from the stimulating effect. Others simply fall asleep.

The problem of cat training lies with the word "training" itself. Cats are never really trained as we understand the word, unless you are talking about the big cats in a circus.

Training is more or less a form of behavior modification where the animal is conditioned to respond to a stimulus, especially when the desired response is outside the animal's usual range of behavior. For example, housebreaking a dog is training because it is natural for the dog to relieve himself anywhere except where he sleeps and eats. A trained dog will only relieve himself outdoors or indoors on newspaper and usually at one prescribed place. In the case of cats, however, it is probably more accurate to use the term "cat management" when describing cat training.

Managing your cat at home does not require the rigors of a complete obedience course as does the management of a pet dog. The following are the only demands you need make on your cat to enjoy a pleasant home life:

1.   Litter box orientation
2.   Come when called
3.   Walking on leash
4.   "Sit"
5.   "No"

Training Techniques

Motivation

No cat can be made to obey because he wants to please you or is terrified of you. It is only on the simplest level that cats accept the dominant/subordinate idea at all. With the exception of lions, cats in the wild are solitary figures stalking their prey in the lonely shadows of a variety of remote regions of the world. The hunt is not always successful, and dinner isn't on the table at five every day. Like their undomesticated cousins, house cats are always in search of food, because they cannot associate that instinct with the fact that you are going to feed them on a regular basis. Cats behave as though these were two separate issues. It is on this basis that humans can manipulate their cats and modify their behavior.

All cats, in a sense, are constantly on the hunt for food, whether they are hungry or not. Consequently they can be trained to obey a few simple commands as long as there is a food reward given in exchange. Bribery is the name of the game, but it is for a higher purpose.

The same basic procedures are followed when training the big cats for the circus. Of primary importance is to get to know the animal personally. This is essentially the bonding process. This means that you must spend considerable time with your cat before starting a training (or management) program. It's important to learn individual peculiarities in order to determine how to motivate and reprimand the cat, and get him to react. The most important thing is to learn the animal's native abilities. Each cat has his own gimmicks for getting what he wants, and these can be useful in manipulating behavior.

Whether taming big cats or training domestic house cats, you can use the *hunger drive* to your advantage. Of course, you must feed your cat the normal diet that is necessary to maintain the animal in a healthy condition. However, for training purposes reduce the ration a bit so that the cat's appetite is sharpened just slightly before each training session. It is probably best simply to conduct training sessions for domestic cats before the daily feeding rather than to reduce the ration. Give the cat a basic diet that he gets whether he trains or not. Then find a food substance that he likes and use it as a supplement to the basic diet. Cats love yeast pills or little bits of cooked liver, for instance. Contrary to what most people think, cats work better when they are hungry. When working a lion or tiger in a show or demonstration, the trainer works it hungry because that's when the trainer is safe. When the big cats are full, they want to curl up and sleep and not be disturbed. The trainer gives them food rewards while they're working (very small amounts) and feeds them when it's over.

The Bridge

When training a cat, start slowly. Get the animal's confidence and take time to give him an opportunity to understand what you want. When teaching commands, you should develop a hand signal as well as a verbal signal plus a clicker, bell, or whistle to serve as a "bridge" between signal and reward. The cat must be told when he's doing something correctly in order to reinforce what he's learned. You start getting him used to the signal or bridge by feeding him the reward and following it immediately with a whistle or a click. It's best always to hand-feed the animal; never put the food in a pan as a training reward. Giving food rewards by hand helps the cat fix on you as the source of his food and makes him come to you for his meals and rewards. In this manner you work with him and get the behavior you are looking for. In many instances the cat will walk toward you and do some stunts and tricks just to get your attention because he wants to be fed. This is perfectly normal behavior, particularly if he's just on the edge of hunger. Don't make the cat too hungry. In that case he won't think of anything but food.

If you use the bridge consistently at the beginning of training, the cat will always associate the sound with the food reward, and this is the first breakthrough in training cats. From there you start working the cat with the behavior he offers or the behavior you want from him. By developing a cat's proper response to a bridge sound you can teach almost anything and expect good results.

Imprinting

The ideal training situation is to have the cat imprint on you from the very beginning of his life. The best results occur when you start talking to the kitten around the fourth day of his life, even before his eyes have opened. You talk to him and caress him frequently so that imprinting on you takes place. Imprinting is a learning process limited to a specific developmental period and one that leads to an extremely rapid conditioning. If the animal focuses on the imprinting object—in this case, you—during this very early or sensitive period, he will always prefer the imprinted object.

The Training Environment

When you are training an animal, it is important to focus all of your concentration on the animal. The training environment must be quiet and offer no distractions for the trainer or the animal. Cats can get frightened quite easily by people coming up behind them, especially strangers. It is important that there be only pleasant associations with the training sessions. It is also worth mentioning that cats work best on their own territory. Do not train outdoors and do not train at locations other than in the cat's home. You must be the focus of attention and the only relief from boredom. Be patient and do not play with the cat during training sessions.

Training Sessions

The cat should be worked every day. The length of each session depends on the attention span of the animal. Because no two animals are alike, you will have to determine this for yourself based on trial and error. Some cats will train no more than three minutes, but can tolerate three or four sessions a day, spaced well apart. There are other cats who will tolerate five-, ten-, and even fifteen-minute sessions, but in this case you should limit the sessions to one a day. In each session continue to work the animal as long as he will work readily. Always stop the minute the cat has performed a command sharply, no matter how short the session was. Do not push him to perform the command again. Always stop the first time he performs correctly and leave him with a good experience and feeling. The next day work him again, and if he performs properly the first time, you can get him to repeat the action once. Do not bore the animal by having him constantly repeat something he has learned to do well.

It is extremely important to understand what to do if the cat becomes panic-stricken for any reason. Never pick up a frightened or panicked cat. Leave him alone, get the area quiet, resolve the source of the animal's fright. Give the cat as much time to settle down as he wants. Even a small kitten can be nothing but a mass of claws and teeth if he is very upset. He has the tools and the ability to rip anyone wide open, exposing people and other pets to infection and the necessity for medical treatment.

Whole tomcats and unsprayed females are not very good candidates for training. It is almost impossible to train a male cat with a strong sexual urge. The same is true for a female during estrus. The management of cat behavior is best achieved when the pet has been surgically sterilized. A physically sick cat is also impossible to work with. Cancel all training sessions until the animal is well. Do not train the cat if *you* are not well, either. Otherwise your techniques may become sloppy, which will certainly carry over to the animal.

Litter Box Orientation

The most obvious functions of the cat's eliminative processes, of course, are digestion, nutrition, and elimination of the body's waste matter. However, there is more to it than that. Cats use their body waste as scent posts for the purpose of marking off territory and also as a means of communicating with other cats. Females in heat and males looking for females mark off areas with their urine to attract each other. In this situation the urine contains glandular secretions that give it a special odor with sexual connotations. Body waste is also connected with health functions. Frequency of elimination and the quality of feces and urine are often indicative of the animal's state of health. Additionally, most cats express their anxiety and negative emotions by eliminating outside of the litter box. All of these factors may be involved in your cat's litter box orientation. Therefore, when your cat suddenly stops using the litter box, it may not be a simple matter of training or spite or anything concerning discipline. A sick or emotionally upset cat will have housebreaking failures. Solving the underlying problem is the only way to get the animal back to using the proper toilet.

For the first two weeks of life the kitten has no physical ability to eliminate on its own. Elimination is accomplished with the help of the mother, who simply licks the underbelly and the genital regions, thus stimulating urination and defecation. She ingests the body waste from the kittens so that no detectable odor comes from the nest. This natural response promotes survival because it prevents enemies and predators from locating the litter by scent. Similarly, her own body waste is eliminated away from the nest and buried. It is for this reason and this reason exclusively that cats instinctively bury their body waste. For the pet owner it is a blessing since a cat's natural proclivity to keep odors to a minimum (with the exception of territorial and sexual marking) makes him the best of pets.

The first three weeks of kittenhood may be compared to the first eight months of a human baby's life. The kitten's eyes open, hearing begins, and just about all physical functions begin to work without outside stimulation. The kitten begins to crawl and eventually gets himself outside the nest for a look at the greater world. It is extraordinary that the youngster has already learned not to eliminate in his own nest. The mother is very strict about this and does not permit it. At this early age many kittens have already begun to travel a relatively far distance from the nest in order to relieve themselves and make infantile digging and burying gestures. All of this works to the advantage of humans who wish to live with cats as companion animals. Assuming a kitten has been with his mother and litter mates for at least eight weeks, litter box orientation is an easy and quick process.

The Technique

Following each meal, after every nap, and after strenuous play, place the kitten (or grown cat) in the litter box and take hold of the front paws. Push them forward and backward so that the cat has to make a scratching motion. On most occasions the instinct to eliminate will take over, although the cat will not always eliminate each time this is done. Do not force the issue. Remember, you cannot force a cat to do anything. Allow the cat to hop out of the box for a few minutes' pause. Do not permit the animal to leave the room. It is advisable to close the door from the outset. Repeat the procedure. Depending on your cat's intelligence, mood, and patience with you, he will eventually give the desired result. The bathroom is the ideal location for your cat's litter box.

Supervision is important. Therefore, never give the cat the run of the house unless you are right there, watching for a mistake. If he sniffs one spot constantly, begins to act fidgety, or scratch the floor or carpet, it's time to transport him to the litter box quickly, close the door behind you, and repeat the front paw scratching motions. Chances are it won't be necessary.

Confinement is a very important aspect of this technique. Keep the cat in the room with the litter box and nowhere else unless he is constantly supervised. Place a dish of water in with him, and perhaps a toy or two. Young kittens need a little time to learn to find the room with the box in it. Even a grown cat may decide to place a scent signal on the far wall of a new dining room simply because he hasn't been patterned to use the litter box yet. Also, kittens may not be able to control their small bladders and sphincter muscles while on the way to the room with the litter box. Very few cats will deliberately soil their living space if they can help it. They are too fastidious.

Confining the cat to one room helps him to pattern his behavior in the correct way by making the litter box more immediately available than any other place in the home. Once a cat soils an area outside the box, he will constantly be drawn back to the spot because of the odor. *Do not let this develop into a pattern because it will be extremely difficult to break.* When the cat makes a mistake, it is important to clean it up and destroy the urine scent as fast as you can. There are several products for sale in pet supply stores and mail-order catalogs designed to eradicate urine stains and odors. Remember, the odor (imperceptible to humans) is the most important signal that you need to eradicate. Purchase a product that refers to itself as an odor neutralizer.

Normally it is essential to keep the litter box clean by scooping it out every day and changing the clay or sand very often (some owners change it every day). However, during the orientation period it is a good idea to leave the litter slightly soiled so that the scent will attract the cat to the box.

Do not neglect or reject the idea of confinement. Even a cat who has always used a litter box should be confined when not supervised at least for the first twenty-four hours after moving into a new home. Continue to confine kittens until you are certain they know what to do and where to do it. It shouldn't take more than two or three days, if that long.

Patience and persistence are the keys to training animals, but when a cat is in poor health or is emotionally upset, he fails to use his established toilet area. When cats fail to follow the dictates of house training, they are either sick or disturbed about something, and those are the issues that must be dealt with rather than training or retraining.

Teaching Your Cat His Name

Cat training really begins by teaching your pet his name. A cat learns his own name by hearing it repeatedly and associating it with something pleasant. One must never use the cat's name for punishment, for scolding, as a way of expressing your anger, or for any negative purpose. The cat's name is useful when you want him to come to you. If the association is negative, no cat (or dog, or child, or employee) will come running upon hearing you call. When teaching your cat his name, dole out a food reward every time it's said, and pet and praise the animal affectionately.

Once the cat learns his name, he is practically trained to "come when called."

A cat that knows his name is a more manageable pet. Teach him his name simply by calling him at every opportune moment. A call to dinner is the most effective time to teach a cat his name. Always offer your cat a food reward when you call him by name, and give him verbal praise and gentle petting for responding properly. When training a cat, you must use a soft, friendly tone of voice. Never punish a cat after calling him to you. That is to destroy his trust.

Come When Called

Now is the time to use the bridge technique. As stated earlier, get the cat used to the signal or bridge by feeding a reward and then creating the sound either from a soft whistle or from a clicker, the small metal type used by children at Halloween (usually shaped like an animal or insect). Feed the cat a small reward and then click the clicker or blow the whistle softly. Always hand-feed—offer the reward from the flat of your palm. Do this five or ten times and quit for the day. Repeat this procedure for three or four days. By then your cat should be accustomed to working with the bridge. As Pavlov's dog salivated at the sound of the dinner bell, your cat should expect a food treat when he hears the bridge and will be willing to repeat the commands you will or have taught him.

The next step is to reinforce the cat's responding to his name. As stated earlier, a cat learns his own name by hearing it repeatedly and associating the name with something pleasant. The cat's name is useful when you want him to come to you. When teaching his name, stand back just a short distance from him while he is on the floor. Say the cat's name, pause for one second, drop a small food reward, pause for one second, click the clicker (bridge). When the cat eats the morsel, tell him what a good cat he is. Repeat these actions five or ten times, but on each occasion take two steps backward so that the cat is following you each time you call him. Give the cat two sessions, half an hour apart, then quit for the day. Repeat this step for three days.

At the next session place the cat in one end of the room and walk to the other. Call the cat by name and add the word "come." At the same time use a hand signal. Start with your right arm hanging at your side, and swing it up-upward and around as though beckoning, so that it touches your left shoulder, then gently return it to its original position at your side. After the execution of the hand signal, click the clicker (bridge). As the cat begins to move toward you, hold out your hand with the food reward sitting on the flat of your palm. Bend forward slightly so that the cat can lick the reward off your hand. As he does, congratulate him. This praise reinforces the food reward. Walk to the opposite end of the room and repeat the procedure. Do this five times if the cat performs well and ten times if he does not. Remember the procedure. Call the cat by name, adding the word "come": "Albert, come." At the same time use the hand signal. Immediately after the hand signal, click the clicker (bridge). Offer the reward on the flat of your palm and then give the praise. Once again, work the cat in two sessions, spaced apart, each day, and do this for three days in a row. Miraculous as it may seem, you have now taught your cat to come when called.

Walking on a Leash

How often does a cat get to enjoy canine prerogatives at a camp fire, munching on barbecued hot dogs after vigorous backpacking? A trip to Yellowstone or even an outing in the building elevator is a pleasure rarely shared by the family cat. For those who enjoy the company of their cats, there is a way to take them almost anywhere. The key to cat travel is the leash and harness. Bear in mind that it is just as unnatural for a dog to be attached to a leash as it is for a cat. The dog makes the adjustment, and so can the cat.

Ideally, leash training is initiated during kittenhood. However, there is no reason why grown cats cannot be trained to walk in tow, if they are brought to it with patience, sensitivity, and intelligence. The correct equipment, while simple, is absolutely essential. Unlike dogs, cats and kittens must not use collars with leashes. To prevent a collar from slipping off over the head, it would have to be buckled too tightly for comfort and safety, and the cat's negative reaction would be a natural one. This is the primary mistake that is often made when trying to walk with a cat on a leash. Instead of a collar, use a cat harness. A well-fitted *figure-eight harness* is best, accompanied by a long, lightweight leash. The leash should be made of nylon or webbed cloth. A leather leash is fine, provided it is six feet long, light yet strong.

The initial problem is getting the cat to adapt to wearing this equipment. Some cats from the very beginning will not mind, while others will resist with obstinate vigor and take a long time to make the adjustment. Start with the harness. Give it to the cat as if it were a toy. Lay it at the cat's feet and allow him to sniff it, move it about and even use it in play. Once he is convinced the harness is not dangerous, put it on. Allow the cat to wear it for the better part of the day; repeat this for two days. It might even be a good idea to place the harness in the cat's bed so that he can claim it as his own "territory."

Next, place the harness on the cat, tie a twelve-inch strip of cloth, rope, or string to the harness, and leave it on for five to ten hours. Do this for two days. Do not encourage the cat to play with the cloth if you can help it. Then hook the actual leash to the harness instead of the cloth strip. This will be a different experience. The greater length and weight will annoy the animal. For the first day do not hook the leash to the harness for more than thirty minutes at a time. If the cat seems receptive, leave it hooked for as long as eight hours. Repeat this for two days.

You are now ready to pick up the leash in your hand and attempt to walk with the cat. It may go well in the beginning when you are both walking in the same direction. The problem begins when you exert just the slightest pressure and turn to walk in another direction. The cat will definitely balk and maybe dig in his paws (or claws), coming to a screeching halt. If he begins to fight the leash, lies down, or seems otherwise disturbed, be gentle and kind, using soft words, and coax him slowly to follow you. Perhaps an offer of his favorite type of food reward will help. Never, never drag him around on a leash; this will simply not produce the desired result. Never assume that your cat will walk like an obedience-trained dog. Walking with a cat is more like a negotiated settlement than the result of a direct command. You both share in the decision as to which direction you will walk.

The moment of truth comes when the cat is to be taken outside for the first time wearing a harness and leash. It is important for you to know that, for the cat, being exposed on the sidewalk is more frightening than the unnatural sensation of being tethered. Hold the cat for as long as you must, even for the entire first experience. Next, kneel and entice him to come to you, using reassuring entreaties and food rewards. Be patient and very sensitive to his emotions. Eventually, the typical, healthy cat will make the adjustment and walk as you walk.

You must be certain that your cat has a suitable temperament for this type of exercise. The very shy, cowering cat, who would rather be home under the bed than anywhere else in the world, is a very poor candidate for leash training. But if your cat is extremely curious, gregarious, and somewhat adventurous, then by all means afford him the pleasure of your company by teaching him to walk with you on a leash. Be prepared to pick him up if a stray dog or other potential threat appears, or you may find yourself serving as an impromptu tree climbed by a terrified cat equipped with eighteen razor-sharp claws.

"Sit" (Sit Up, Jump, Down)

The objective here is to get the cat to sit where you want him to, even if that means getting him to jump onto a chair or stool. Once the cat is seated, it is easy to get him to rise on his hind legs for you and then, on command, to leap back to the floor. This is not as difficult or as complicated as it might seem. You will simply employ the same principles of training as before. The sound bridge made with the clicker is important here because it is the link between your command and the cat's desire to be rewarded. For this reason it is important that the cat be somewhat hungry before and during the training sessions. As stated before, conduct the sessions before meals.

At the start of the session, work the cat in the manner described in the "Come When Called" section earlier. Once he comes to you, give him a food reward, immediately followed by a click (the bridge). Kneel down slowly, keeping his attention on you by staring in his eyes. Say "Sit," gently push his hind section down into a sitting position, give him a food reward, click the clicker, and offer him lavish praise. Repeat this five times and then quit. Conduct another session one or two hours later, doing the whole thing over again. Repeat this each day until the cat will sit on signal, without your having to push his rear end down.

The next step is to get him to jump onto a chair or stool and sit for you. While the cat is at one end of a room, set up a stool at the other end. In a friendly but firm voice say the cat's name, followed by "come." Don't forget to use your hand gesture. When the cat gets to you, kneel down and give him a food reward. Click the clicker immediately and praise him. Then say, "Sit." If he sits for you, give him a food reward; immediately click the clicker and praise him. Rise to your full height and hold out a food reward with your hand halfway up the length of the stool. The cat will probably try to reach for it while still in a sitting position. Say his name and "Jump." If he starts to get poised as if he is going to jump, place the hand holding the food reward slightly above the height of the stool so that he must aim for the stool as a landing ledge in order to get at the reward. Allow your arm to slide up and down (like a trombone) so that the reward is an enticement for the cat to jump onto the stool. When he finally makes the jump, give him the reward instantly and click the clicker just as quickly. Praise the cat. It is important that the food reward be given immediately after he performs properly so that he associates the command with the reward. It is equally important that the bridge (the clicking sound) and the praise come instantly after the food reward is given, for the same reason. Repeat this sequence of stimulus-response-reward five times and then quit. Conduct another session one or two hours later and repeat the procedure. Do this for several days, until the cat is performing the command sharply.

The next and final stage is to get the cat to come when called; sit; jump onto the stool, sit, and jump down. Repeat the three steps, as above. When the cat gets up onto the stool and is given his reward for doing so, give him the command "Sit." He should respond readily. When he does, give him a food reward immediately, click the clicker, and praise him. Let him remain seated on the stool for fifteen seconds. Hold out a food reward in your hand, down near the floor (using the same trombone movement as before). Say the cat's name and "Down." When he jumps down, kneel and instantly give him the reward, click the clicker, and praise him. Repeat this five times, then quit. Repeat the procedure one or two hours later. Repeat this lesson every day until the cat is performing it with precision. It will not take too long.

Tricks

The question of cat tricks is a matter of your personal taste and preferences. Teaching your cat to perform tricks can be another way to bond with your furry friend, to exercise him, or simply an opportunity for fun and games. Tricks are not very difficult to teach; it's a matter of observing what the animal likes to do on his own and then encouraging him to perform when asked. For example, many cats enjoy rolling over. If you can catch him in the act, give him a food reward, click your clicker, and praise the animal. If you say "Roll over" every time the cat is about to do it, then reward him for doing so afterward, he will eventually roll over on command. The same applies to shaking hands, jumping on your shoulder, and retrieving, as well as the dubious feat of begging.

Cat tricks are merely the formalization by humans of various behavior and individual quirks that some cats manifest automatically. Some cats' principal talent may be not bolting away when facing a group of people. It is a rare quality in a cat and should be rewarded.

Some cats never perform tricks no matter how hard you

try. They may be unwilling or simply not as intelligent as other cats. Some cats will learn to perform instantly while others will take a much longer time to develop the behavior pattern. For you to accomplish anything with a cat requires that you have a relationship with each other. It is all much easier when you know your animal and he knows you.

A famous circus lion tamer, Gunther Gebel-Williams, said in an interview with me, "You have to be always strong. You command animals with your presence. They must respect you. Without respect, it is all over. First you must find an animal and it must learn its name. Then you have to wait until it is old enough to begin training. When you begin training you must be patient. You need to take time and in animal training, one year is nothing. It is all a matter of communication. It is all in your voice, your touch and in your personality. You must maintain the authority of your personality. When I say I feel very close to my animals, it's not only words. If I miss a morning with them, I feel bad. I do everything I can for them. If they are cold I cannot rest. They are like my family."

Cats do not stop loving their owners if the owners decide to take control of their behavior. In fact, it strengthens your rapport with your pet. Having a well-trained cat is a happy circumstance for both four-legged and two-legged inhabitants of any household.

7

CAT PROBLEMS

Cats are not always angels and sometimes behave in ways that are upsetting to people. Here, the troubled cat owner will find some solutions for the most common cat problems. Perspective, however, is an essential part of finding solutions that work. Review the information detailed in Chapter Three, "Cat Scan." This will help you understand the difference between *behavior* and *misbehavior*. With few exceptions, a working knowledge of the information offered in Chapter Three will help you understand why the cat is misbehaving and set the stage for creative problem solving beyond the solutions offered here.

Many cat owners stumble around for years with the behavior problems of their pets, hoping that they will disappear as if by magic. When they don't, the owners either learn to live with the problem or, unfortunately, get rid of the cat. The solutions to feline behavior problems offered in this chapter are meant to get the cat owner started on the right track. Through trial and error cat owners must try to find their own solutions when those suggested here do not work. The answers to pets' problems can be as different as one cat is from another. The same problem may have to be solved ten different ways for ten different cats. What works for one may not work for another. Pet owners should begin tapping into their own imaginations, getting rid of that helpless feeling, and start relying on their own instincts and creative energy.

Assuming the relationship with your cat is important to you, the solutions for these behavior problems require effort, patience, and understanding. You should evaluate your cat's behavior as normal or abnormal—for a cat. On occasion a pet will seem to behave strangely, but its behavior, which is probably inherited or instinctive, may be absolutely correct for a cat, despite the fact that it conflicts with what is acceptable to you. What is required of the pet owner is a knowledge of basic cat behavior, so that elements in the environment that stimulate unpleasant behavior can be changed, eliminated, or at the very least, understood. If a cat's behavior is abnormal when compared to its true nature, there is little chance of effecting change without help from a trained animal expert. Fortunately, most feline behavior problems can be solved by adjusting the living conditions that created the problem or by employing one or two simple behavior modification tactics.

When a cat behaves in a manner that is disturbing to humans, such as peeing on the floor, or making a mad dash through the living room, or destroying your possessions, something may or may not be wrong. The disturbing behavior may either be caused by the expression of a basic instinct or by some negative factor in the environment that is upsetting the cat. For example, if a cat has a need to roam and that need is thwarted, it may do some damage in the house. The damage may be done not to spite you, but perhaps as a result of trying to get out. The cat may be scratching the window curtains or woodwork on the door in an attempt to get out. When a cat has an overpowering need to get out of the house (perhaps to respond to a female in heat), he may damage your home. But this must not be misinterpreted as the cat's having a destructive or spiteful nature. A cat may simply be responding to his needs. This is part of being a cat and must be understood and accepted as such by the cat's family.

"No!"

Much of your cat's negative behavior can be stopped and eventually changed with the help of the demand "No!" Although the word should be said in a firm tone of voice and with assertion, it must not be used as a reprimand or as a punishment. It is, rather, a tool for stopping the cat from doing something unacceptable. Of course, there is a suggestion of reprimand when you say "No" to your cat in a firm tone of voice. When used properly, "No" will stop the cat from whatever he is doing. It is invaluable for maintaining discipline and having things your way.

This term is essentially a negative one and is associated exclusively with discipline. Many of the cat behavior problems mentioned throughout this chapter require its use. Cats *can* be disciplined, and the sooner this is accomplished the better life is going to be for everyone. The object is to stop unwanted behavior before it becomes generalized or habitual without rhyme or reason. All cats develop patterned routines of behavior. If the family is patient, consistent, and loving, those behavior patterns can be pleasing and appropriate for the human environment.

The cat must be caught in the act if he is going to stop his bad behavior, no matter what it is. Bear in mind that each time you use the demand "No," you are not only stopping unwanted behavior in that instance, you are also conditioning the cat away from future misbehavior. A loud noise or a sharp "No" will get his attention and signal your displeasure. Most cats hate loud, sudden noises and will do almost anything to avoid them.

"No" must be said with precision, which is to say that no other word or term or phrase should clutter the demand. Do not add any other word to the demand or you will dilute its impact for future use. Also, the word must never be used for anything except stopping the cat from continuing an unwanted action. This is crucial.

How to Use "No" as a Problem-Solving Tool

When your cat misbehaves and you catch him in the act, you may use "No" in two ways:

1. Keep a water pistol handy and squirt it at the cat (not in the face) and say "No" in a loud tone of voice; slap your hand loudly or stamp the floor with your foot. By startling the cat, you will create a negative association with his misbehavior. Do not make any extreme gestures that could be interpreted by the cat as a threat of violence. Fear will get you less than nothing with a cat.

2. Grasp the cat by the nape of the neck, pick him up, holding him out in midair as you support his bottom feet with your other hand, and shake him firmly. At the same time, say "No" in a firm tone of voice so that there can be no mistake about your meaning. Do not shake the cat too hard. This is the manner in which the mother conditions her kittens. "No" can be administered in this fashion for all unacceptable behavior and can be used for healthy cats of all ages.

In a short period of time only the verbal use of "No" will be necessary to stop your cat from unwanted behavior.

Redirected Behavior

It is not enough to stop your cat from doing something wrong. You must also teach him what he *should* be doing instead. To change your cat's behavior pattern on a permanent basis, you must *redirect* his behavior to something or someplace else that is acceptable to you *immediately following your firmly stated "No."* For example, if your cat scratches your furniture, say "No" as suggested earlier and carry the furry offender to his scratch post. Gently squeeze the front paws until the claws show and rub them into the material, allowing the cat to get the feel of scratching in this acceptable place. Then praise the cat and give him a small food reward. You have stopped the cat from the unwanted behavior, showed him where you want him to do it, and rewarded him for doing it there. That is the entire process as it must be executed if it is to be effective. The idea is to teach the cat what to do by conditioning him rather than just giving reprimands.

It is absolutely essential that the teaching portion be reinforced with food rewards and loving praise immediately following the redirection. The rewards and praise reinforce the teaching/conditioning process. There can be no permanent result without the reinforcement. The cat will work for the food reward until the desired behavior simply becomes a habit or patterned behavior, making the food rewards unnecessary.

House Soiling

Of all the problems cat owners face at one time or another, house soiling is probably the most upsetting and perplexing. Urine or feces deposited outside the litter box is unsightly, offensive, and totally unacceptable. A cat may urinate or defecate on the floor, the carpet, the bed, or in the bathtub.

Assuming your cat has been using his litter box properly for a while and suddenly starts eliminating on the floor, it is essential to understand what is causing the problem in order to solve it.

It Could Be a Medical Problem

Some cat owners may not be aware of the fact that misbehavior is often caused by illness. A cat that is not using his litter box may be sick and should see a veterinarian, if only to rule out a medical problem. For example, it is common for male cats to develop feline urinary syndrome (FUS), which involves inflammation of the bladder and urethra and the formation of urinary stones and plugs, causing obstruction of the urethra. Signs of this condition are frequent attempts to urinate and straining to urinate, with possible traces of blood in the urine. Immediate medical attention is necessary, as this illness can be life-threatening when not treated in time. A cat suffering from FUS will continually try to urinate outside his litter box. It is most common in male cats and especially male cats that have been altered. *Incontinent behavior can also be a sign of various other illnesses. See a veterinarian.*

It Could Be a "Territory" Problem

The most common reason for house soiling is cats "spraying" or marking territory with urine as a means of claiming it. Please refer to "Territory" in Chapter Three, "Cat Scan" for an understanding of the role of body waste in claiming territory. It is also useful to read "Litter Box Orientation" in Chapter Six, "How to Train Your Cat." Male cats that are not castrated will back up against a vertical surface such as a wall or door and spray a stream of scented urine against it. The purpose of this is twofold: to claim territory and to attract the attention of a female in heat. Females and castrated males will also use urine for this purpose, but they may stand and spray or use the squatting position. The most common solution available for this is surgical neutering. Having your male or female cat sexually altered may or may not solve the problem entirely, but it will certainly reduce its intensity.

It Could Be an Anxiety or Emotional Stress Problem

This is the most common reason for cats not using their litter boxes. Cats that are emotionally upset will suddenly and without warning soil the floor (or the bathtub) with their urine and defecation. It is an expression of their emotional state. Many things can upset a house cat, but a major cause is permanent change in the family routine. A death in the family, divorce, kids going off to college, going on vacation and leaving the cat home, or any other drastic change in the cat's life can cause emotional stress. Here are but a few of the important events that upset family cats:

Acquiring a second pet. Adding a dog or a second cat to your household may cause your resident cat some emotional stress resulting in house soiling (or aggressive behavior). This is a common response but should not be tolerated for long.

Allow the new animal to walk freely into the situation. There may be some hissing and spitting along with raised hackles, but this will soon end. The best situation is when two or more cats begin their lives together as kittens. The same is true of a puppy and a kitten. The next best situation is when the newcomer is a kitten (or a puppy) and the cat in residence is older. This gives the cat with seniority a definite advantage in terms of claimed territory and physical dominance. There may be a brief fight about who is top cat, but it won't last long and shouldn't be allowed to get violent. Within hours or a few days at most the senior cat should get over any house soiling problems. If not, try giving the newcomer a separate litter box of his own as far from the older cat's established territory as possible, as well as separate food bowls and feeding locations. If the two animals become embroiled in prolonged, intense hostility, they will have to be separated temporarily or perhaps permanently. The original resident must always be given first consideration of attention and territory. One or both animals may have to be put in a cage or separate room. Leaving the cage door or the door to the other room open allows them to gradually and carefully investigate each other and come to some peaceable settlement.

Moving. Next to losing its family, there is no greater cause of anxiety in a cat than moving to a new house or apartment. It is all connected to the importance a cat places on his territory. Moving away from their territory creates a traumatic shock for most cats. When first entering his new home, the cat's instinct is to mark it in several places with his urine and/or feces as a way of claiming the area as his new territory. It is almost impossible to prevent this from happening. However, have the litter box placed at a location convenient for you but never near the front door or window, to prevent the cat's running away. Teach the cat to use the litter box all over again, as if he had never been trained. See "Litter Box Orientation" in Chapter Six, "How to Train Your Cat."

Sensing one or more strange cats close by. Occasionally a house cat will see another cat from the window roaming into his territory. In some instances the cat will see or even smell a strange cat from a slight opening beneath the front door. This is very upsetting to most cats and will cause them to soil outside the litter box and in the area close to the door. The house soiling is most often a form of scent marking as an assertion of territorial possession. (This is not usually a problem in a multi-cat household.) Another negative response to sensing a strange cat is to refuse to use the litter box if it is too close to the intruding cat. That is another reason for not placing the litter box near the front door or window.

Actions You Can Take if Your Cat Is House Soiling

1. Keep the litter box clean. Cats will not use it if it is saturated with urine and feces. (This is also a matter of good hygiene as well as preventive medicine.) Scoop the solids out of the sand once or twice a day and replace the sand entirely once or twice a week.

2. Try changing the brand of litter in the box. Some cats prefer one texture over another, such as sand as opposed to clay granules. Some cats develop an aversion to the deodorizing chemicals in certain products.

3. Once your cat has expressed his need to claim territory by marking the floor with the scent of his urine and feces, you must eliminate the odor from those locations thoroughly. Use a high-quality odor neutralizer meant for this purpose. This will help prevent the cat from returning to the same places and remarking them. Odor neutralizers are sold in concentrated liquid form or in aerosol spray cans. They can be purchased in pet stores and through mail-order catalogs specializing in pet supplies. Do not use store-bought ammonia for this purpose. Ammonia is an ingredient present in urine and has the opposite of the desired effect by attracting cats rather than repelling them.

4. Give your cat extra play time and loving attention.

5. If you catch your cat in the act of house soiling and he does not respond to your verbal demand "No," squirt him with a water pistol (not in the face) and say "No" in a firm tone of voice. Eventually, just saying "No" in a firm tone of voice will suffice.

6. If the cat is soiling the bathtub, try keeping one or two inches of water in it for a while.

7. Retrain your cat. Refer to "Litter Box Orientation" in Chapter Six, "How to Train Your Cat." Retraining may require confining the cat for several days to a small room or cage with his litter box in it. This will encourage the cat to use the box instead of the floor. Slowly increase the area the cat is allowed in.

8. In a multi-cat household try maintaining one litter box for each cat.

9. Have your cat surgically altered. This means that males are neutered (castrated) and females are spayed (ovariohysterctomy).

10. Use your ingenuity. If your cat, for example, persistently returns to the same spot to urinate on it, cover it with a piece of furniture so he cannot re-soil it. Take him to his litter box whenever he goes near the spot. If your cat backs up against your front door and urinates on it because he can smell or see another cat from the outside, do the following: Find a way to discourage the presence of the strange cat and eliminate your cat's ability to see or smell it. This could involve the use of manufactured cat repellents in addition to sealing up cracks at the bottom or sides of the door. Be innovative.

Scratching Problems

Most new cat owners are concerned about their cat's insatiable desire to scratch the furniture, the curtains, the carpeting, and just about anything else he can get his claws into, including parts of your body. This can be a serious behavior problem considering the cost of new furniture or medical attention.

As detailed in the "Territory" section of Chapter Three, "Cat Scan," a cat marks territory or communicates his presence all too often by clawing visible scratches into a vertical object such as a tree, if you're lucky, or the arm of a sofa, if you're not. This is instinctive behavior and is almost impossible to eradicate. Although clawing has to do with leaving visible scratch marks of assertion and territorial marking, the most important reason for it is your cat's physical need to remove the outer sheath of his claws.

Your Cat's Claws

Feline claws are unique because they are retractable and are not seen when in their retracted position. When cats walk, only the very tips come in contact with the ground. The claws are formidable weapons and are extended when the cat prepares to fight, run, or climb. The claws are also unsheathed when the animal is frightened or panicked. Unsheathed claws are necessary for catching prey animals. The claws are also necessary for climbing, executing escape maneuvers, playing, fighting, mating, and other activities. They are *indispensable,* causing many cat lovers to discourage the medical procedure of *declawing,* which is the surgical removal of the nails by a veterinarian to avoid scratching problems. Declawing is really an amputation of the digits, comparable to removing fingers, not just the nails. For that reason no declawed cat is allowed to compete in cat shows officially sanctioned by national registry organizations such as the Cat Fanciers' Association. Serious cat breeders and exhibitors emphatically discourage pet owners from having their cats declawed. A declawed cat cannot defend itself or catch prey animals. It cannot climb, run fast, or jump with precision and grace. The Cat Fancy considers a declawed cat to be unnatural or deformed. Most pet owners who have had their cats declawed considered it the last best chance for their cats to live with them. It is a major controversy among cat lovers. You are urged not to declaw your cat unless it saves him from losing his home.

How to Avoid Scratching Problems

Scratching problems must be eliminated as soon as possible, preferably in kittenhood. It helps if the kitten is able to watch his mother use a scratching device designed for cats. The owner must also help. Take any kitten or cat to the scratch post, gently squeeze the front paws until the claws show, and rub them into the material until the kitten gets the feel of pulling on the object with his claws. The scratch post must be sturdy enough and tall enough for the animal to reach up and stretch out on it without tipping it over.

A twelve-inch post may be a nice toy for a kitten, but you'll find that it's useless as a substitute for your furniture. Scratching is an important physical behavior for your cat and cannot be stopped. The trick is to *redirect* the cat's need to scratch, to an acceptable object, so that it is no longer a behavior problem. The answer is obvious. Obtain a suitable object for your cat to scratch on and condition him to use it exclusively.

Every cat needs something designed especially for him to scratch. It could save you hundreds of dollars by avoiding damaged furniture, carpets, curtains, clothing, and other possessions. Cats develop behavior patterns early in their lives that are difficult to change. Unless you set the proper pattern of behavior quickly, your cat is going to scratch whatever is handy and appealing. In all likelihood it will be your furniture that is damaged. Once the problem begins, it is hard to stop.

Disposable scratch pads. Many experienced cat breeders use disposable scratch pads made of corrugated cardboard. This convenient product is usually imbued with catnip and is very appealing to cats. A cardboard scratch pad is a rectangular product, approximately eighteen inches long by six or ten inches wide, that lies flat on any surface. Place your cat or kitten on top of the pad and allow him to get his scent on it so that it becomes his possession. Hold his front paws and move them up and down along the rough surface, initiating scratching motions normal for a cat. Few scratching problems ever develop when this technique is employed early and often. Once the scratch pad is torn beyond recognition, simply throw it away and replace it. They cost under ten dollars.

Scratch posts. Most permanent scratch posts are vertical pieces of wood anchored to a flat base and covered with carpet, canvas, or burlap. Cats will gladly use them instead of your furniture *if they are high enough* and if they are appealing. Your cat must reach the top of it with his front claws when standing on his hind legs. There is nothing more useless than a scratch post that is too short. An effective scratch post can simply be a log lying horizontally or leaning vertically against the wall if it is secured to the floor. Other posts are made of cork or loose fabric of all kinds. Try rubbing catnip into it or attaching a small rubber ball at the top with a string. Do anything that will make the post attractive to your cat, so that he will use it instead of your furniture.

(Rubbing the scratch post with catnip is only effective once the animal is past five months of age. Cats do not seem to respond to catnip until they begin to mature sexually. Some neutered cats never respond to catnip.)

Cat furniture. These imposing, somewhat expensive objects are designed for cats to scratch and play on as well as use as a high territory perch. They come in many sizes, shapes, and types and have some kind of covering that is meant for cats to get their claws into. The more expensive pieces are tall (as high as nine feet), elaborate treelike structures with carpeted platforms and covered enclosures forming a kind of feline playground. Although they are costly, they are highly desirable to cats and their owners who enjoy watching them. All cats take to them immediately. They are advertised in every cat magazine, available in most pet supply catalogs, and often displayed by vendors at cat shows.

Teaching your cat to use a scratch post. This should be done on a daily basis and as often as possible. When you find the animal scratching anyplace other than the post, you must discipline him and then show him what is the acceptable thing to do.

Hold your cat by the nape of the neck, pick him up, hold him out in midair with the bottom feet supported by the flat of your other hand, and shake him. At the same time say, "No" in a firm tone of voice so that there can be no mistake about your meaning. Do not shake the cat too hard. This is the manner in which the mother chastises the kittens. It is perfectly acceptable as well as effective. The command "No" can be administered in this fashion for all unacceptable behavior and can be used for adult cats as well. If your cat runs away before you can discipline him in this manner, try using a water pistol or plant sprayer from across the room accompanied by your firm "No."

Eventually, saying "No" in a firm voice will suffice, without the shaking or the water pistol. Consistency is very important. Once you begin disciplining with "No," always use that word exclusively for that purpose and no other. In that way the word becomes an effective training tool. Say it in a loud and resonant voice.

Create an aversion to your furniture. This is accomplished by simply covering the areas of the furniture that your cat abuses with thick sheets of plastic so that it is unpleasant and dissatisfying for scratching purposes. Affixing snapping mousetraps to areas that are covered with several thicknesses of newspapers will scare the cat when he sets them off without hurting him. Balloons serve the same purpose.

Stick a pin in a blown-up balloon next to your cat in order to startle him and create an aversion to the large, inflated sphere. Then tape several blown-up balloons to the damaged area of your furniture. The sight of them may be enough to keep the cat away. Certainly, if the cat pops one, it will create the desired aversion.

Trim your cat's nails. When a cat claws a scratch post or your furniture, he is responding to an important physical impulse to remove the outer layer of nail and make room for the continuously growing, sharper layer underneath. Much of the damage to yourself and your possessions can be avoided by keeping the nails trimmed. Your cat's nails should be trimmed at least once a week.

How to . . . The idea is to put gentle pressure on each nail so that it extends out of the skin covering just for clipping. Place the cat's paw on your open fingers with your thumb on top. Select the nail that needs trimming and press your thumb on top of the corresponding toe. The nail will appear. With the nail trimmer in the other hand, cut the nail.

Nail trimmers for cats are specially designed and *nothing else* should be used. These vital tools are readily available in a pet store or mail-order catalog. If the nails are a quarter inch past the pink area, they should be clipped. Most cat nails are white or buff-colored at the tips and pink as they get closer to the base. The pink area is called the *quick*; it indicates where the nerve endings are located and where the blood vessels begin. *You must never clip the nails at the quick to avoid hurting the cat and causing him injury.* If you trim the nail just at the curve, you will avoid any problems. If the procedure is too nerve-wracking for you, take the cat to a groomer or veterinarian and observe the professional's technique.

Once the nails have been clipped with the cutting tool, it is a good idea to smooth down the sharp edges as you would when cutting your own nails, with an emery board and nail buffer. Some cat owners use the emery board exclusively as a way of keeping the nails in trim. This procedure is an important method for preventing scratching problems.

Coping with the Damage

A new kitten or cat can make your home look like a marked-up subway car in less than a week. Any cat is capable of destroying carpets, upholstery, floors, furniture, and walls by scratching, chewing, playing, mischief-making, and of course, uncontrolled body eliminations.

You may not be able to totally control your cat's destructive behavior, but you can spare your home from the unsightly results of it. It is possible to preserve your home and your possessions with pet-proof decorating. It is a matter of decorating with materials and products that can stand up to the potential abuse of normal pet behavior.

The most serious problems are on the floor. At times cats have litter box failures, in addition to sometimes getting sick all over your floors or carpeting. This can permanently stain expensive carpeting. Scrapes, scuffs, and scratches are a common floor problem from your cat's sharp nails. You need a floor that can withstand the worst animal assault on it and still look good. Your best options are a first-rate wood floor, permanently waxed vinyl or urethane floor covering (newer forms of linoleum), or one of the new stain-resistant carpets.

If you decide on easy-to-clean wood floors, seriously consider oak (sanded and finished) because of how well it wears and looks. You could also choose prefinished laminated wood flooring because of its resistance to moisture. Check under your carpet. You may already have a wood floor that could be restored. A hard finish on your floor will definitely withstand any abuse your cat can dish out. If given enough time to cure, the finish will resist your pet's digging, scratching, and soiling.

A good floor covering for pet owners is vinyl or urethane sheets or tiles. Old-fashioned linoleum is not as good because its felt backing causes moisture damage to the floor beneath and because it does not stand up to serious wear and tear. Once upon a time nonporous floor coverings were found only in kitchens and bathrooms. But now the incredible selection of sophisticated colors and patterns have made it possible to use them in almost any room in the house.

Sheet vinyl offers the advantage of an almost seamless surface, although vinyl tiles can be installed by anyone, especially if they are self-sticking. All you do is peel off the paper backing to expose the adhesive, place the tile on the floor, and press down firmly. Such a floor will give you an important advantage when dealing with a cat who often coughs up hairballs. Many of the leading manufacturers of vinyl and urethane floor coverings have a no-wax feature with stain resistance, gloss retention, and resistance to abrasion. Staining is not much of a factor with the no-wax vinyl so long as the mess is not allowed to remain on the surface for a long time. Urethane, however, offers a tougher, more scratch-resistant surface than vinyl.

There is also an answer for those who prefer carpets or rugs. Stain-resistant carpets have made it possible to have your cake and spill it too. Special fibers in stain-resistant carpeting protect floors from most household stains, and that includes whatever your cat can come up with. You are better off selecting tweeds, tone-on-tones, and pebbled textures to help hide dirt and lint. Patterned designs on stain-resistant carpets help enormously.

If your pet stains your furniture, look for a stain-proof fabric protector label the next time you buy an upholstered chair or sofa. Stain-proofing that is applied at the mill is your best chance for resisting pet stains.

Aggressive Behavior

Few people think of cats as being aggressive, unless they have endured the pain of a deep puncture wound from a cat's teeth or the tearing of skin from his claws. Cats can be as menacing as dogs or any other species. Still, only a few cats are aggressive toward humans. Some researchers believe that because cats do not include humans as part of their social order of rank, they do not normally express aggression toward them. It is a fact that most aggression in domestic cats is directed toward other domestic cats (and their prey).

If you consider the larger cats in the wild and then think of the domestic cat as a smaller, tamer version, it is not too difficult to imagine a house cat that is unfriendly and even dangerous.

Although the domestic cat physically resembles the smaller wild cat, it is related to *all* the wild felids and their fierce behavior. There is some unique behavior among the various species of wild cats, however, such as the tiger's ability to swim and its nomadic existence and the leopard's cleverness at fooling the animals it hunts and its ability to climb trees, where it often eats what it has captured. The greatest difference among the great cats, of course, is the lions' *pride,* which is a group structure they live in, unlike the solitary existence of the other species. Nevertheless, most of the behavior of cats is similar, including that of the domestic house cat.

Solving aggressive behavior problems is not only beneficial for the cat's family, it is equally important for the cat's state of health. Aggressive behavior can be a symptom or a cause of physical and emotional stress. Cats that are in a constant state of stress may experience a decrease of appetite or various digestive problems which will prevent the body from obtaining essential nutrients. Cats in stress have lower resistance to disease.

Aggressive Behavior Toward Other Cats

Aggression toward one another among domestic cats is predictable in some circumstances and not in others. For example, cats that live with other cats are usually well adjusted and tolerant of their fellow felines and share the space peaceably. Those that are accustomed to being the only cat in the family are most often intolerant of other cats entering their territory, especially on a permanent basis.

When cat meets cat. Cats may become aggressive (or soil the house) when a new cat is introduced into a single-cat household. Aggressive behavior is most often the outcome when free-roaming males meet each other, outdoors. They will fight for territory, superior rank, mating privileges with a female in heat, or for combinations of the three.

It is difficult to persuade a cat that has established his territory as the sole feline resident in your home to accept a new cat. Typical responses from the established cat are to ignore the newcomer, sulk and hide, spray a wall with urine (or relieve himself on the floor), or provoke a fight with the intruder. In most cases, the cats eventually come to terms with each other and make an adaptive adjustment. In some cases the problem is never resolved and one or the other cat must be found a new home.

Aggressive behavior related to sex. Male cats are violently combative if they must compete for the attention of a female in heat. During the time that a female goes into her estrus cycle, most available males in the area can smell and hear her condition. If they are allowed to roam freely, they will congregate around her and go through the ritual of mating. Territory is violated, and the rules of social rank must be decided by serious fighting among the males. While the female waits for the outcome, the available tomcats assault one another for top-rank position.

There is much that is violent about sexual encounters between feral cats or cats that are allowed to roam through their own neighborhoods. (Matings arranged by serious, knowledgeable breeders of purebred cats are very different. There is no violence in those situations because there is only one male and one female for the mating.)

Male versus female. In other situations involving aggression, male and female cats will fight with each other over matters pertaining to their territorial rights. Almost all females become extremely aggressive when defending their young from males, females, or other species of animals, including humans and dogs.

Aggressive Behavior Toward Humans

Defensive aggression. Aggressive behavior toward humans is usually exhibited when a cat perceives danger to himself. Most cats that bite humans do it out of fear. When a cat perceives that he is cornered, he will take a defensive posture and lash out with his claws and teeth. Most cat bites are defensive in nature, although not always justified or appropriate. Once the cat believes the threat is gone, he ends his hostile behavior and almost never pursues his adversary. This behavior is also displayed against cats and dogs that are threatening.

Pain aggression. Another cause of aggressive behavior is pain. If you hit a cat or pull at him or hold him in an inappropriate manner that causes pain, he will scratch or bite you. This frequently happens to children who pull a cat's tail or grab his fur with clutching fingers.

Love bites. One of the more perplexing forms of feline aggressive behavior is a cat biting during or after he has been stroked or petted in a loving manner. Some cats hold a part of your hand firmly but gently between their teeth as you pet them, but they inhibit their bites and do not break the skin. Some investigators have concluded that this bite is similar to the *nape-bite* that is used by males to hold females in position during copulation.

Play aggression. When this form of aggression is directed toward humans, it is seen as hiding, stalking, and sudden pouncing, usually at the human ankle. It is a behavior most commonly indulged in by kittens as a form of learning and practicing for their future as adults. If this behavior is not corrected and redirected to appropriate toys, it will become generalized and seen throughout the life of the cat.

Aggression caused by disease. Aggressive behavior in cats directed at humans (or other animals) may be caused by the pathology of various medical conditions such as tumors in the brain, constricted blood vessels in the brain, rabies or toxoplasmosis (a parasitic disease caused by the protozoa *toxoplasma gondii*). A normally well-behaved, gentle cat that becomes unusually aggressive, especially toward humans, should be examined, tested, and diagnosed by a veterinarian.

How to Cope with Aggressive Behavior

Using a simple correction for most situations. Cats that display aggressive behavior must be disciplined and conditioned away from it. When cats or kittens scratch, nip, or bite, they must be corrected, as described earlier, in the following manner:

Take the misbehaving cat by the nape of the neck, pick him up, hold him out in midair, support him by placing the flat of your other hand under his hind legs, and shake him. At the same time say "No" in a firm tone of voice so that there can be no mistake about your meaning. Do not shake the cat too hard or he will always fear you. This is the manner in which the mother chastises the kittens. It is perfectly acceptable as well as effective.

The "No" can be administered in this fashion for all unacceptable behavior and can be used for adult cats as well as kittens. If your cat runs away before you can discipline him in this manner, try using a squirt bottle or water pistol from across the room, accompanied by your firm "No."

Eventually, saying "No" in a firm voice will suffice without the shaking or the water pistol. Consistency is very important. Once you begin disciplining with "No," always use that word exclusively for that purpose and no other. In that way the word becomes an effective training tool. Say it in a loud and resonant voice. It is extremely important that you then pet your cat and speak lovingly to him for having stopped his misbehavior. This should be done after the correction. You may even give him a small food reward, providing a small space of time has passed and it cannot be misinterpreted as a reward for the bad behavior.

Segregating cats. When cats become aggressive toward each other in a multi-cat household, it may be necessary to separate the offending cats in different rooms or to place one or both in cages or cat carriers to avoid harmful fighting. Feed the cats in their cages or carriers at opposite ends of the same room. Each day the cages or carriers should be moved closer together. The idea is that the cats will be fed only when they are together. This should establish the association of food as a reward for accepting each other's presence. When the cages or carriers can be side by side without any signs of aggression, the cats are ready to have the run of the house.

Medical therapies. When the aggressive behavior of a cat is intense and all other measures have failed, try consulting a veterinarian. If the cat's problem is defensive aggression or poor socialization and is based on fear, the vet might suggest treating with tranquilizers such as diazepam (Valium).

If the cat's aggression is based on assertions of territory or dominance over other cats, the vet might suggest treating with progestins, which are female reproductive hormones that sometimes reduce aggressive behavior.

Aggressive behavior can be prevented by having young male cats and kittens castrated by a veterinarian. Castration is a surgical procedure that has, in some instances, modified the aggressive behavior of adult male cats. Castrated males are less likely to roam far from home since they are not stimulated by females in heat. Having had their sex drive eliminated, castrated males are also less likely to initiate fights with other cats. Although surgical neutering is not guaranteed to abruptly stop aggressive behavior, it does modify it to some degree. Of course, the primary purpose of castration is to prevent producing unwanted kittens, which impact on the pet overpopulation problem.

Eating Problems

Refusing to Eat (Anorexia)

When a cat stops eating, it may not be a matter of being finicky about food. Cats that refuse to eat may be suffering from emotional stress caused by any of the problems discussed in this chapter. In addition, some cats cannot or will not eat when they are placed in a strange environment, such as a boarding kennel or hospital. *Inappetence,* or refusing food, is often caused by fear, depression, anxiety, or worry.

When a cat refuses food on a continual basis, it could be a sign of a medical condition requiring immediate veterinary attention. Anorexia can be related to wounds of the lips or oral structures, infection, abscess, fever, metabolic disorders, intestinal obstruction, injury, tumors, or just about any disease state. Anorexic cats are vulnerable to various medical problems of a serious nature that are related to nutritional deficiencies. Veterinarians may treat this condition with various appetite stimulants and tranquilizers, vitamin therapy, or in extreme medical situations, with forced feeding by tube.

Finicky Eating

Change in the diet is the most common reason for a temporary decrease in appetite. It can also be caused by various
emotional states, ranging from fear to excitement. Because
weight loss follows quickly, along with vulnerability to
disease caused by nutrient deficiencies, the problem should
be dealt with immediately. Feed the cat foods and delicacies that are appealing, such as *small* amounts of cooked
organ meats, cooked fish, cantaloupe, or whatever seems to
stimulate his appetite. Then reintroduce the old diet that the
cat prefers. Once he is eating again, wean him away from
the old diet and introduce the new one. This is accomplished by feeding three-quarters of the old ration along
with one-quarter of the new ration. Each day take away
one-quarter of the old food and replace it with one-quarter
of the new food. In four days the cat should be eating the
new food in a normal fashion.

To determine your cat's food preference, consider what
his basic diet would be if he were on his own in the
wild. Such cats live on mice. All cats are carnivores and
prefer meat, although they do eat small amounts of grasses,
cereals, and fruits when in the wild state. Feed your house
cat some form of muscle meat on a frequent basis and keep
the diet varied so as to avoid "addiction" to any one type
of food, such as liver or fish.

Overeating

Obviously, the result of eating too much is obesity, which
is usually damaging to the animal's health, resulting in a
shortened life span. In addition to the unsightly look of
obesity, it is also implicated in diseases of the heart, res-

piratory conditions, kidney failure, osteoarthritis, damage to the digestive system, diabetes, infections, and rendering a cat a poor risk for surgery.

Obesity is caused by three factors:

1. Endocrine disorders may cause an animal to gain more weight than his frame was meant to hold. These and other medical dysfunctions creating obesity must be treated by a qualified veterinarian.

2. As a cat grows older, his ability to metabolize food decreases along with his energy output. Despite this metabolic reduction, the quantity of food given (and eaten) is often the same as it was when the animal was younger. The result is obesity.

3. The third cause is so simple that few believe it: Overfeeding. When the cat's caloric intake exceeds his energy requirements, fat is created and stored in the body. This is the most common explanation for obesity in cats (and dogs, and people). The only way for a cat to lose this excess fat is to eat fewer calories daily. If the cat is given fewer calories than he needs, he will draw from his own fat deposits around the body to create the needed energy. That requires putting the cat on a diet. Consult a veterinarian or simply reduce the amount fed by 25 to 50 percent. Another option is to use one of the diet rations for cats that are available on the shelves of supermarkets everywhere.

It should be noted that there are certain stages throughout the life of all cats when the need for nutritional intake is greater. These include pregnancy, lactation (nursing kittens), the maximum growth stage of kittenhood, and when working cats live in colder regions. Older cats have different nutritional needs, including reduced caloric intake. Consult a veterinarian or purchase commercially prepared food formulated for older cats.

Never, never, never feed a cat food that was formulated

for dogs. Dog food does not contain the quantity of protein and fat necessary to maintain the cat's health.

Obsessive Chewing, Licking, and Sucking Behavior

The most common of this behavior is the inappropriate mouthing of objects in the environment. Wood may be chewed, plastic materials licked, or fabrics such as wool sucked until they are destroyed.

There is speculation among behaviorists and other investigators about the root cause of this peculiar and perplexing activity. Wool or fabric sucking and some forms of chewing are attributed to premature weaning, especially among Siamese and Burmese breeds. It may be related to feeding in some way, such as a desire for the roughage normally supplied by grass and other plant materials. Abnormal chewing and sucking behavior may also be the result of boredom, loneliness, lack of attention, or some form of emotional problem.

There are only two workable solutions here. You can either deny the cat access to the textured objects he is obsessed with or you can modify his behavior with corrections and redirection. See "No!" at the beginning of this chapter.

Eating Poisonous Plants

If a cat jumps into a rosebush, it's bad for the roses but it's worse for the cat because of the thorns. A short-haired cat walking through a patch of nettles is on shaky ground, as he will probably have tremors and twitches by the end of the day, caused by the liquid injected by the stinging hairs. When our beloved fauna tries to eat our beloved flora, the flora can fight back. Whether your cats are indoors or outdoors, they are vulnerable to the harmful effects of some plants.

What do Japanese yew, mountain laurel, lily of the valley, philodendron, dieffenbachia all have in common? They are beautiful to look at but potentially toxic to pets, children, and even to adults. Although plant poisoning is uncommon, small animals and young children can find themselves in a life-threatening emergency if they nibble on plants such as these.

However, it would be a great disservice to those who love the refreshing beauty of natural greenery to advise them to ban *all* such plants from their homes. Instead, it is useful to know which plants are potentially harmful, in order to prevent accidents.

Toxic plants must be eaten in sufficient quantities to produce the effects of poisoning. The toxic dosage varies with the species of the plant, the stage of plant growth, the part of the plant consumed, the soil type, and other environmental factors. Harmful dosages are also affected by the animal species in question. Children or dogs may be less susceptible to a given plant poison than a cat or a bird, based on body weight.

It is fortunate that cats do not depend on foliage as a staple in their diets. In most situations, they will eat only a small quantity of the offending growth, with little or no reaction to it. Most cats eat grass and then regurgitate it. This behavior may relate to the animal's need or desire to cleanse his digestive tract. Many pets that nibble away at plants do so out of boredom or curiosity. Other factors involved in plant eating are the age of the animal, the feeding habits of the owner, and new or altered surroundings.

Poisonous plants may affect the mouth, throat, esophagus, stomach, intestines, nervous system, blood and circulation, heart, or brain (altered behavior, hallucinations). The signs may be mild, such as lack of energy, or intense, such as digestive upsets, or extreme, such as depression, coma, and death. When such signs are apparent, it is important to consider plant poisoning as a possibility if the animal has been exposed to toxic growths.

Poisonous plants affecting the mouth, throat, and esophagus with irritation, ulcers, excessive salivation, or swelling (sometimes interfering with breathing) are dumb cane, philodendron, caladium, skunk cabbage, and Jack-in-the-pulpit. Plants affecting the stomach and digestive tract with either irritation, vomiting, nausea, depression, abdominal pain, diarrhea, possible fever, coma, or death are amaryllis, daffodil, tulip, and wisteria bulbs; English ivy, alfalfa, beech, daphne, iris, bird of paradise, box, crown of thorns, euonymus, honeysuckle, poinsettia, castor bean, precatory bean (rosary pea), black locust, nightshades, Jerusalem cherry, and potato (green parts and eyes).

Those affecting the cardiovascular system are foxglove, lily of the valley, oleander, monkshood, larkspur, cherry pits, peach pits, apricot pits, almond pits, apple seeds, and hydrangea.

Plants affecting the nervous system with either trembling, irregular heartbeat, abdominal pain, nausea, vomiting, salivation, convulsions, thirst, alterations in behavior, dilated pupils, or sudden death are Japanese yew, English yew, Western yew, American yew, Indian tobacco, golden chain, mescal bean, poison hemlock, tobacco, rhubarb (leaves, upper stem), belladonna, henbane, jimson weed, jessamine, datura, periwinkle, chinaberry, coriaria, moonseed, water hemlock, marijuana, and morning glory.

Among dangerous plants, the least considered or understood are those that are "mechanically injurious." Mechanical injuries involve those plants that either irritate, lacerate, or puncture the skin. Contact irritants or mechanical injuries can be produced by nettle, nettle spurge, stinging nettle, bull nettle, burdock, blackberry, cactus, Carolina nightshade, foxtail, goathead, honey locust, needlegrass, sandbur, tripleawn, wild barleys, and wild bromes.

The list of plants potentially dangerous to pets is, indeed, a long one. A few general principles should be remembered. First, get the poisonous material out of the animal. Take the plant away if the animal is "caught in the act." Contact a veterinarian immediately for instructions.

What to do when your cat eats a poisonous plant. When plant poisoning does occur, it may be a life-threatening situation requiring fast action if your pet is to survive. Take the following steps:

1. Try to determine what the poisonous material was, when it was ingested, and the amount swallowed.

2. Call your veterinarian or nearest poison control center. Inform your veterinarian of the animal's age, any medical problems, if he is taking medication, and whether or not he has vomited.

3. If possible, bring the poisonous material to the veterinarian with the animal. The sooner you get professional advice, the better the chance for survival. Remember, plant poisoning is rare, but poisonous plants are not.

How to prevent plant poisoning. Keep poisonous plants hanging out of your pet's reach, or in a separate room that is off limits to animals. As the spring gardening season approaches, bear in mind that outdoor plants can carry chemical poisons. Highly toxic herbicides and organophosphate pesticides on grass clippings can also be deadly.

In order to break the habit of chewing on house plants, you can sprinkle red or black pepper on the leaves and at the base of the plant as well as in the soil. Cats are very intelligent and will not repeat an action that causes them immediate discomfort. Because all cats first sniff what they eat, the pepper will be inhaled and cause a great deal of uncomfortable sneezing. If a cat actually eats or licks the pepper, he will not like the hot taste that is waiting for him. You can also place a grid of chicken wire over the surface of the soil. Cats that climb potted trees may be discouraged by placing around the trunk a homemade collar such as those used on ship tie lines to repel rodents.

The best thing is to provide cats with something they can and will eat, so their natural needs are provided for. At the same time make house plants less attractive with the use of the pepper as a repellent. When given a choice, cats will be more attracted to grassier things. Grow wheat grass in a pot specifically for your cat to eat. A pot of wet, moist soil with some wheat grass seed spread on top will come up in a couple of weeks. This will give you a plant that your cat will usually prefer to almost anything. Wheat grass is cheap and can be obtained at a health food store.

Disturbing Nocturnal Activity

Whenever a new cat owner discusses the furry blessed event of the family, the subject of strange nocturnal behavior comes up. It's quite predictable. It is often referred to as the "Midnight Special," but others have called it the "Midnight Crazies." It is usually described something like this:

"Late at night, after we've all gone to bed and are in a sound sleep, we hear a sudden crash. It could be a lamp falling over or the trash can tipping to the side. Out of a cloud of dust comes the thundering sound of hoof beats as the feline night stalker races across the entire house, up one wall and down the other. The cat stops high atop the highest point it can climb and lets out a chest-beating MMRRROWL at the top of its cat's voice and then begins its run again. Only this time it runs sideways, stops in the middle of the room, leaps straight off the ground, and pounces down with all its might. It goes on for ten minutes. When the dust settles, we try to get some sleep . . . unless the cat starts it all over again."

Kittens, young cats, and even some older ones are remarkably playful. This behavior seems to peak in the middle of the night with a high energy spill. No one seems to know why it happens. It is a secret shared among cats. Those who must clear the wreckage in the morning can only guess about it.

This behavior often begins with a full use of the litter box, offering the possibility that it has something to do with reaffirming territorial rights. Cats claim territory by marking it (litter box scratching, clawing the furniture) and vocal proclamations that sound like lion roars in the middle of the night.

We can only guess about why this behavior is displayed late at night. For practicality's sake, perhaps, since this is when cats have the run of the house without interference. They sleep most of the day and appear to have what can only be described as an overflow of energy at night, when they become lively (after the family has gone to bed). According to feline behavior researcher Dr. Paul Leyhausen, "Events almost always happen at night. This is not because the cat is predominantly nocturnal, but rather because the animals dislike being observed and are sensitive to noise and commotion."

The other irritating nighttime activity is play behavior. Although cats are not truly nocturnal creatures, they are very well equipped for darkness. They see better in dim light than most mammals and can make sound hunting decisions based on their keen sensory abilities. Some researchers believe that cats, like owls, recognize ultraviolet rays given off in darkness from the bodies of some animals. Their response to the subtle vibrations caused by prey animals plus their remarkable hearing capacity make them keen night hunters.

It is all too common for kittens and even grown cats to make a routine out of play rituals in the middle of the night. Play is practice of prey-catching techniques, hunting methods, fighting behavior, escape behavior, sexual activity, and simply for exercise and fun. The feline technique for hunting is to stalk and ambush, utilizing maximum energy in an instantaneous rush of bursting effort as they pounce on their prey. This behavior is mostly practiced when cats play, especially at night when no one is observing them. Domestic kittens habitually use even more energy in play than they would when actually hunting. It is little wonder, then, that their nocturnal behavior tends to keep their families awake. Worse yet, the play can become destructive to possessions and property. Garbage pails, lamp cords, books, magazines, clothing, all should be placed out of harm's way before retiring for the evening.

Excessive nighttime play occurs when the owner does not actively initiate play behavior or when the cat is always confined within small quarters. This is especially true for kittens and young cats.

A Possible Solution

Provide more opportunities for a variety of play activities during the day and early evening hours to help the cat express its excess energy. Tossing a crumpled piece of paper around as if it were a ball can be quite interesting to a cat. Ping Pong balls are among the feline favorites. Play should be both interactive between cat and human and solitary when the cat wants to be uninterrupted. Solitary play should involve toys that cats can play with themselves such as wooden thread spools, balls, and various kinds of squeak toys. A companion cat or other animal such as a dog is a possibility if one can be found that is compatible with your family cat.

One way to cope with a nocturnally active cat is to confine the animal to one room for the night. The best place is where the food, water, scratch post, and litter box are located. The only problem with this is the cat's anxiety. Some kittens and adult cats will adjust to being confined in one room alone for the evening and some will not. You can choose to confine your pet in your room if you do not mind its sleeping with you in the bed.

With the nocturnal overflow of energy, we see all aspects of hunting and prey capture. The "cat crazies" involve sudden dashes across the room in a crouched position, stalking, a watching posture, creeping, pouncing, seizing with the teeth, carrying around, and tossing objects away. To the novice cat owner this is a startling and perplexing set of behavior. But it is harmless, fascinating, and more often than not, quite funny if not outright lovable. The best adjustment is to accept it as a fact of life.

Coping with Your Cat's Desire to Catch Mice

Part of keeping your cat happy is understanding his needs and behavior and somehow allowing for it. Possibly the least understood and most criticized aspect of cat behavior is how they deal with mice.

Most people believe there is something sadistic about the way cats catch and ultimately kill mice, birds, flies, or anything else they can capture. Once they catch a mouse, they appear to enjoy tormenting the poor, hapless rodent, who must succumb to the cat's seemingly bizarre behavior.

After a cat catches a mouse, he moves it from place to place by holding it in his teeth. The cat will set it down and look at it. When the mouse begins to run, the cat chases it and snatches it from the ground with its teeth, only to move it to another location. After several awful minutes the mouse, bless his soul, stands up on his hind legs and flails at the fascinated cat. It is a heroic drama with a sad, inevitable ending.

Once again the mouse is carried away in the cat's mouth and neatly placed at the feet of just about anyone in the human family. The cat then looks this way and that way, yawns contentedly, and bites the mouse on the nape of the neck. Once the mouse is dispatched and lies motionless on the ground, the cat pushes it with his paws, in what appears to be an effort to revive it. The intrigued cat may even toss the little body in the air. Once the cat understands that the mouse is dead, the sad little drama has reached its conclusion.

Sooner or later your cat will present you with a peculiar gift—a dead or dying mouse. What is it about a cat and a mouse that so entwines their destinies together? They are like cops and robbers, Holmes and Moriarty, Tom and Jerry. Only they play for keeps and the outcome is not funny.

Why do cats have this need to give members of their human family dead mice? It is a fact that the cat and mouse are natural enemies, and it is a safe assumption that they have been at one another since prehistoric times. Both species will eat just about anything, including one another. However, cats feed largely on rodents when on their own. What brings the cat and the mouse together is the shared relationship of predator and prey, nature's love-hate relationship.

For most who witness the confrontation of the cat and

mouse drama, it would appear that the cat is the villain, exercising cruelty and meanness of spirit. Cats are not cruel, mean, or unfeeling. They are simply one of nature's creatures responding to impulses elicited by the natural behavior of their prey. Cats are among the most competent hunters in the animal kingdom and mice are what they hunt best. It cannot be changed. Both creatures are genetically programmed for this relationship.

The Tom and Jerry chase is really about food. For whatever arbitrary reason, cats regard mice as a movable feast. It is a dispassionate hunt for a meal that sets the scene. Cats instinctively respond to the sight, smell, and movement of mice (some insects, birds, and larger rodents too). The instinct to stalk, chase, capture, kill, and eat mice is very powerful and is usually in operation whether the need is there or not. The drive for prey capture is overwhelming. Cats chase mice whether they are hungry or not, because of their incredible drive to survive, despite the fact that most of them never eat what they capture.

Although most cats will chase a mouse, only those who were taught by their mothers will deliver the killing bite on the nape of the neck. There is a misconception that cats play with their fallen prey because they are mean and sadistic. This behavior is genetically programmed into their catalog of behavior so that they will teach kittens about catching mice by eliciting unused instincts. If nothing else, throwing the mouse about certainly captures the attention of otherwise inattentive kittens, preparing them for lessons in survival. Both males and females possess this behavioral trait.

Every finely developed skill the cat possesses serves in the hunt for mice and other sources of food. No other animal has evolved into such a virtuoso hunter as the cat. The cat's keen vision, quiet manner, agility, and flawless leaps are all part of his great hunting ability. His desire to sit high up, to play at night, to chase a ball of yarn, to scratch the carpet are all part of a secret rehearsal to ambush and capture, to kill and eat. Try to imagine your cat living alone on the Serengeti Plains like his larger cousins. His hunting behavior would seem more acceptable then.

Oddly enough, there is little need for all of this, what with the incredible selection of manufactured cat food available in supermarkets everywhere. But try and explain that to your cat.

By the way, the reason cats present dead mice at your feet is simple. They are attempting to teach us about catching, killing, and eating them. They possess an instinct to bring to a litter of weaning kittens live mice so that their newly learned play behavior can translate into a methodology for survival. Every kitten has the instinct to chase and capture a mouse. But the lethal bite on the nape of the neck must be taught by an adult cat (usually but not always the mother) along with the idea that mice are a source of food. Most cats have this teaching instinct even if they never have kittens, and it is not restricted to females. Some males and even some neutered males will attempt to teach members of the human family how to be good mousers by bringing the captured animal to them. In this respect most cats behave like inspired English teachers directing the school play.

When your cat presents you with a freshly caught mouse it is wise to express your appreciation rather than run away. You may dispose of the "gift" after your cat leaves the room.